LEARN TO UNDERSTAND AND SOLVE YOUR SLEEPING PROBLEMS

Analyze your sleeping patterns by using the Sleep Questionnaire and Calendar inside.

Consider the multitude of factors influencing a good night's sleep.

Review the causes and types of insomnia; learn what sort of person sleeps better than others.

Find out the techniques and medications that are supposed to help you sleep relaxed.

Discover the one natural sleeping pill found in many foods.

THE INSTANT SLEEP METHOD

**WE HOPE YOU
ENJOY THIS BOOK**

IF YOU'D LIKE A
FREE LIST
OF OTHER PAPERBACKS
AVAILABLE FROM
PLAYBOY PRESS,
JUST SEND
YOUR REQUEST TO
MARILYN ADAMS,
PLAYBOY PRESS,
919 NORTH
MICHIGAN AVENUE,
CHICAGO, ILLINOIS
60611.

the Instant Sleep Method

L. Aquino, M.D.

PLAYBOY PRESS

THE INSTANT SLEEP METHOD

Copyright © 1976 by Ventura Associates. All rights reserved. No part of this book may be reproduced, stored in a retrieval system or transmitted in any form by an electronic, mechanical, photocopying, recording means or otherwise without prior written permission of Ventura Associates.

Published simultaneously in the United States and Canada by Playboy Press, Chicago, Illinois. Printed in the United States of America. Library of Congress Catalog Card Number: 76-43397. First edition.

Books are available at quantity discounts for promotional and industrial use. For further information, write our sales-promotion agency: Ventura Associates, 40 East 49th Street, New York, New York 10017.

Contents

	Introduction	vii
1.	*The Question of Sleep*	1
2.	*Sleep, Sweet Sleep ... What Is It?*	11
3.	*Dreaming*	21
4.	*A Full Night of Sleep*	28
5.	*Sleeping Styles*	35
6.	*You Are a Clock!*	44
7.	*What Affects Sleep?*	52
8.	*Insomnia—Man's Universal Malady*	59
9.	*Imaginary or Pseudo-Insomnia*	65
10.	*Situational Insomnia*	71
11.	*Emotional Insomnia*	85
12.	*Voluntary Insomnia—The World Is a Marathon*	93
13.	*Drugs and Drug-Dependency Insomnia*	96
14.	*The Instant Sleep Method—One Step to Sleep*	108
15.	*The Alpha-State—Mastering Your Mind*	115
16.	*The Cloud of Sleep*	120
17.	*The Electric Dormitory*	128
	Bibliography	135

Introduction

Insomnia has always been a topic of interest—poets write of it, physicians suggest cures haphazardly, philosophers dwell on it. As any sufferer can tell you, it is not a pleasant experience. It is a lonely feeling when one lies in bed in the middle of the night trying to clear the mind of trivialities while refusing to consider the day's trials and tribulations... only to realize that the brain has out-tricked the will and is racing about from one thought to another.

There are as many types of insomnia and reasons for it as there are methods of treating it. The first step in curing the malady is to understand why you are plagued by it. You must, with the aid of this book, analyze your personal problem—which will not exactly duplicate the situation anyone else is or has been in. Then you can forge on and actively do something about it. Old habits must be changed, and relearned. There is work and concentration involved with the cure of insomnia. If you are willing to put forth a small measure of time, and will follow my directions, you will sleep. And your whole outlook on life will be brighter.

A great deal of scientific research has been conducted in the area of sleep. We humans appear to be the only insomniacs in the Animal Kingdom. Clearly, part of our problem has to do with the tensions of modern living,

Introduction

as well as other modern environmental situations. We will delve into this also; and you will emerge a happier, more rested, alert person who really enjoys crawling into bed for a night of restful, peaceful slumber.

1

The Question of Sleep

In order to help you cure your sleep problems, you must have a clear understanding of *how* you sleep and what factors affect your sleep patterns. The following Sleep Questionnaire should be filled out as completely as possible. You will constantly refer to this list of questions and answers as you read about my method, and attempt to apply it to your own individual situation.

Some of the questions will stump you. You'll be surprised that you do not know the answers. Try to notice your habits for a few days and you will immediately have deeper insight into your insomnious difficulties.

The sleep Calendar comes first. It is an important part of the Questionnaire. Fill in the day-related queries prior to bed and try to complete the rest as soon as you arise in the morning, if possible.

SLEEP CALENDAR

NIGHTS* 1st 2nd 3rd 4th 5th 6th 7th 8th 9th 10th

1. Number of hours lying in bed
2. Actual hours slept at night
3. Actual time spent catnapping during preceding day
4. Total number of catnaps during preceding day
5. Actual time spent resting (but not asleep) during preceding day
6. Total number of rest periods during preceding day
7. At what time did you crawl into bed?
8. If you awoke during the night, how many times?
9. What time did you awaken in the morning?
10. Did you have alcoholic beverages after 7:00 P.M.? How many?
11. Did you drink coffee, cola, or tea after 7:00 P.M.? How many?

* These records must be kept for ten *consecutive* nights.

The following questionnaire is to be filled out after you have completed the calendar. Jot down answers below each question.

SLEEP QUESTIONNAIRE

1. Add the number of hours you lay in bed for the ten consecutive nights recorded in your Calendar, and divide by ten. This is the average number of hours you lay in bed per night.

2. What is the average number of hours that you actually were asleep? (Calculate this the same way as above.)

3. What is the average amount of time per day that you catnapped?

4. Calculate the average number of catnaps you took within the span of one day.

5. How much time per day did you spend resting, but not catnapping (sleeping)?

6. How many periods within one day were spent resting, on the average?

7. How many times in the average night did you awaken?

8. Do you seem to go to bed at about the same time every evening?

9. Do you sleep with curtains and shades drawn, or in a bright room?

10. Do you have the radio on as you go to sleep?

11. Does a radio or alarm awaken you in the morning?

12. Do you set an alarm or radio to awaken you in the morning but usually wake up prior to the signal?

The Question of Sleep

13. Can you calculate what time you seem to awaken in the middle of the night most often (first, second, or third quarter of the night)?

14. When did you first start to have trouble sleeping?

15. Do or did your parents or siblings have insomnia? Do your children (if applicable)?

16. Do you know whether you were a "good sleeper" as a newborn?

17. If you awaken in the middle of the night, how long does it take you to fall asleep again?

18. Did you sleep well when you were a child? During the teen years?

19. Do you sleep alone? Did you sleep alone when you were young?

20. Do you have a good memory?

21. When is the last time you slept completely through the night?

22. How often do you sleep all night?

23. Do you feel well-rested when you awaken in the morning, or are you groggy for a period of time?

24. Do you get your mind in gear as soon as you awaken, or are you in a cloud until you have a cup of coffee or a shower?

25. Do you immediately hop out of bed in the morning, or do you lounge in bed for a period of time? If you do lounge, about how long does it take for you to be fully awake and out of bed?

26. How much exercise do you get? Do you seem to sleep better when you have exercised during the day?

The Question of Sleep

27. Do you dream? Every night? Rarely? Never?

28. Do you dream the same amount now as you have throughout your life? If not, when did the change take place?

29. As you begin to fall asleep, do you feel as if you are dreaming?

30. When you cannot sleep, what do you do?

31. If you read when you cannot sleep, how long does it usually take you for you to fall asleep again, if you do?

32. When you dream, do you usually dream about recent events?

33. Do you ever have nightmares? About how often?

34. Do you dream in black and white, or in color? Both?

35. When was the last time you can remember going to sleep, and sleeping throughout the night, soundly and without interruption?

36. Do you ever get mixed up as to what is a dream and what is happening when you are awake?

37. Do you take drugs to help you sleep?

38. If yes, how long have you been doing this?

39. Do the drugs seem to help?

40. Do you sleep *soundly* after you have taken drugs?

41. Do you dream when you have taken drugs?

The Question of Sleep

42. What is your usual reaction to drinking alcohol? Does a small amount affect you, or can you consume a great deal without feeling "high"?

43. Do you ever drink to help you sleep? How often?

44. Did you have trouble sleeping when you were pregnant (if applicable)?

45. When you are depressed, do you have more trouble getting to sleep, and staying asleep?

46. What do you usually do before retiring? Watch T.V.? Shower? Read?

47. Do you eat or drink prior to bed?

As you answer these questions, you are gaining insight into your sleep habits and problems. These are the same types of questions sleep researchers compile as they study the sleep quirks of various segments of the population. As you read about my methods to enable you to sleep more soundly and comfortably, the answers you have written in the Questionnaire will facilitate our getting to the root of your particular, personalized problem.

2

Sleep, Sweet Sleep... What Is It?

Sleep is not a simple phenomenon; there are numerous depths and levels of slumber. When you rest, your whole body takes part in the process. There are fine distinctions between your actually being asleep and being on the edge, whether ingoing or outgoing.

The information now available on sleep patterns has been the result of years of research. There are scientists who specialize in sleep; they study and write scholarly reports on nothing else. Often they are biologists, sometimes chemists, psychiatrists, biophysicists, psychologists, anthropologists, and sociologists, who specialize in sleep research. Because of the number of different scientific disciplines interested in the study of sleep, the accumulated data about sleep, while vast, is often difficult to correlate and analyze. There *is* useful, factual data within all the research papers, and when it is brought together and studied, the individual insomniac and his or her problems are more clearly understood, and solvable.

When a sleep scientist sets out to work, the rest of the world is getting ready for bed. Hamlet's lament (Act III, Scene II) that "some must watch while some must sleep," could have been written with a lonely sleep researcher in mind.... The researcher heads for a specially-equipped cubicle within a research institution, hospital, or university. It is late at night. There is a volunteer awaiting the scientist's arrival.

The volunteer is asked to sit down and converse with the scientist about rather mundane, boring subjects. This helps ready the subject for the experiment, which for the volunteer merely means falling asleep. Prior to the subject's retirement, however, the researcher attachs numerous electrodes to the sleeper's body and plugs them into a data-collecting machine. The scientist then enters a second room, often equipped with a one-way mirror.

One would think that the subject might find it hard to go to sleep in a strange place, with someone watching through a window, as cords tangle around. But, amazingly, there is usually no problem. The subject soon closes his eyes....

Prior to the 1930s, sleep researchers had a terrible time conducting their studies. Whenever they attempted to examine their sleeping subject closely they would wake him or her up! All sorts of methods were used: when they carefully pried open the eyelid of the sleeper to discover the condition of the pupil or tried to take a blood pressure reading, it never failed—everyone kept awakening.

They even tried to study themselves. Obviously, it is *hard* to study yourself at sleep because you are asleep and cannot do the studying.

These problems were partially solved after the 30s.

At that time measuring via brain-wave devices was developed, and sleep researchers began to better understand the phenomenon of sleep.

Perhaps it would be truer to say that the scientists found out what sleep *is not*, rather than what it actually *is*. We now know, for example, that a person who appears to be asleep—eyes closed, deep breathing, lack of movement—might not be. Yet the individual who is breathing irregularly and shallowly with a rapid heartbeat might, in fact, be sleeping. This is not our usual image of the sleeper.

Actually there are two types of sleep which occur during every period of slumber. All animals seem to experience these two kinds of sleep—and they have been measured via the eyes, the heartbeat, the brain, and the muscles.

One easily-observed example of these two types of slumber can be found in the family cat or dog. Have you ever seen a household pet lying as though dead to the world, completely lifeless, with eyes closed and breathing deeply? Then a moment later, the animal will be twitching, breathing fast; a moment later slowly, with whiskers twitching and tongue flapping about? The assumption is that Ruff is dreaming. In actuality the animal has gone from one type of sleep pattern into another.

The two types of sleep were discovered rather accidentally by a University of Chicago student, Eugene Aserinsky. It is easy to observe the eyeball moving through the closed eyelid. There is a second way to monitor the movements of the eyeball—with electronic instruments. A Chicago scientist was intrigued by the eyeball's rolling under the lid during sleep and started to measure the movements to determine their relationship to the length and depth of sleep. He gave the chore of monitoring these movements to the student, Aserinsky.

Now these eye movements were thought to be present at the onset of sleep, before the person had succumbed to the depths of slumber, and again would appear as the sleeper began to awake. During deep sleep, the brain was thought to be at rest and quiet; there was no reason why one's eyeballs should be darting about as if the sleeper were watching an exciting hockey game.

Yet our young student found that this was in fact true. Not only were these rapid eye movements present while the subject was fast asleep, but the movements were quicker than could be manipulated while the subject was awake! These findings were totally unexpected and were looked upon with skepticism at first. Yet as Aserinsky monitored with his instrument, and also actually sat next to sleeping subjects all night to observe the eyeball racing around, he realized that he had made a discovery which would change the direction of sleep research. It appeared that not only was the brain not at rest during sleep, but it was in fact *more* active during slumber than during the awake hours of the day.

As research continued, another student, William Dement, found that there were definite relationships: the quick, darting eye movements always seemed to occur as a change in the kind of breathing pattern was noted. Also studies of brain-wave data indicated that there were significant differences in brain activity during the period of rapid eye movements.

It was then realized that sleep was not a resting, quiet condition continuing during the full period of sleep but an alternation of two distinct, recognizable patterns of sleep known as REM and NREM. The term "REM" sleep was given to these periods during sleep when there were specific physiological changes. REM stands for "rapid eye movement," which was the original characteristic of this type of sleep noticed by the scientists. The opposite of REM sleep is termed "NREM" (pronounced non-REM) slumber. NREM sleep is referred to as "quiet sleep" because the body remains still, breathing is slow and regular, and brain activity is minimal. Although the body does not move during NREM-sleep periods, it could. It is not paralyzed, but it simply has not been told to move by the resting brain. During the NREM times, an individual's senses are not working: they are not sending messages to the brain about their environment. The sleeper is out of touch with all that is going on around him or her. If, in fact, the subject does roll over during NREM, there is evidence to indicate that for a moment the sleeper has come out of NREM sleep and will perhaps fall back into it after the roll-over is completed. Thus, NREM sleep is a nonmoving slumber. However, although NREM sleep is called "quiet sleep," it is during this period that snoring occurs, not during the closer-to-wakefulness REM slumber.

Some researchers think that perhaps REM sleep is not actually sleep at all! This "active sleep," say some, is really a period of wakefulness during which the person is paralyzed and hallucinating. During REM, snoring stops and breathing—regular and deep during NREM—becomes short, irregular, and shallow, and at times breathing stops completely for a number of seconds.

Within the REM-sleep phases are smaller segments

of activity such as individual eye movements and twitching of various muscles. Also in REM sleep there are changes in the muscular activity of the middle ear. These REM ear activities are the same as the muscle action which takes place when the ear, during awake periods, "hears" sounds. In other words, when in REM sleep the ear reacts to sound as it does during nonsleep periods.

Both REM and NREM sleep take place during a night of sleep for all humans. The beginning of sleep is usually experienced by the individual as a feeling of floating and sometimes falling. Often this feeling is ended by a jerk which wakes up the rester. During the first few minutes of what we call "sleep," there are several of these episodes of falling sensations followed by a jerking; these episodes are called myoclonias. Although we all experience myoclonias, nervous people seem to experience them more often than others.

Researchers state that the difference between being asleep and awake is that when you are sleeping, you are unaware of your surroundings and when awake, there is cognizance of the environment. The onset of sleep is determined by the exact moment when a person will no longer react in the usual manner to a sound or voice. Of course, if the sound is loud enough, the sleeper will respond—she or he will be awakened!

Scientists who study the phenomenon of sleep have an interesting way to discover the exact onset of sleep. They place a bright light in front of the subject's eyes. They then tape an electric switch to her finger and she is told to press the switch whenever the light is flashed. Then the subject is put to bed—incidentally, a sleepy person is always used for this experiment—and her eyes are taped shut. This all seems very simple. One would assume that the subject will press the switch as she sees the light flash, and that she could not possibly miss seeing the flash. Yet what actually happens time and time again is that the subject will press, and press again, until one time when the light flashes, she will not signal that she has seen it. When the individual is questioned as to why she did not press the signal when she saw the flash, she will be surprised and state that she saw nothing. This is true. At one second, she was alert and responding to light with the press of a finger and the very next second she was unaware that the light flashed, or that she was to do anything about it. She was, in essence, blind—and asleep.

When the precise moment is reached that the subject fails to respond, her eyeballs start drifting slowly from one side to another. This first phase of sleep is always NREM sleep. The depth of the sleep is determined by the amount of stimuli necessary to awaken the sleeper.

The different levels or depths of NREM sleep can be seen on an instrument that picks up brain waves. It will show distinct patterns for each different level of sleep as the sleeper goes under deeper and deeper. What is called NREM Stage One takes several minutes; then NREM Stage Two follows for approximately five minutes. After ten minutes of NREM Stage Three, NREM Stage Four, sets in. It is during Stage Four that it is very difficult to awaken an individual. If one tries to wake a young child during its Stage Four, it will take several minutes, if indeed the youngster can be aroused successfully at all. During Stage Four sleep, children have nightmares and wet their beds. During a nighttime of sleep, this is the soundest sleep of all. If one is prone to talk in one's sleep or to sleepwalk, one will do so at this time.

It takes about thirty to forty minutes to reach Stage Four sleep, which is the deepest NREM sleep. One would think that the next stage would be REM sleep, but it is not. Just as the sleeper went through the four stages of NREM sleep, she must come out of them, step by step, in the opposite direction before she can go into REM sleep. That is, she will go from Stage Four to Stage Three, then Two, followed by Stage One. This second period of Stage One sleep occurs approximately one hour after sleep began. It is followed by a period of REM sleep.

These cycles continue all night long, for all of us. We begin by going through the four stages of NREM sleep, then go backward out of them, and finally we have a REM episode. This is followed by NREM Stage One, then Two, and so forth, again. It takes an average of ninety minutes to go through one of these NREM-REM cycles, so that the eight-hour sleeper goes through about five or six of these cycles each night. In the early hours of sleep, the NREM periods are longer and REM periods short, but as the night wears on, longer REM periods begin and a pattern of shorter NREM periods establishes itself.

If you sleep about seven to eight hours a night, you will experience one to one-and-a-half hours of REM sleep. If you are awakened during a REM period, you will always recall a dream, so we can assume that you dream about every ninety minutes all night long. You have several short dreams at the beginning of the night's sleep, with longer "features" during the deepest hours of the night, followed by some "shorts" at the end of the night's slumber.

Since it is during REM sleep periods that your brain functions, your eyes move rapidly as if you are seeing

Sleep, Sweet Sleep ... What Is It?

The tracings an encephalograph, or brain-wave-measuring instrument, produced during the different sleep-periods, and while awake:

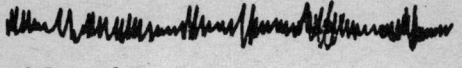

While awake

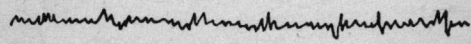

Stage One, NREM sleep

Stage Two, NREM sleep

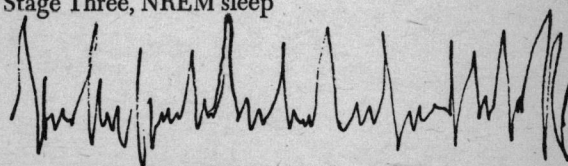

Stage Three, NREM sleep

Stage Four, NREM sleep

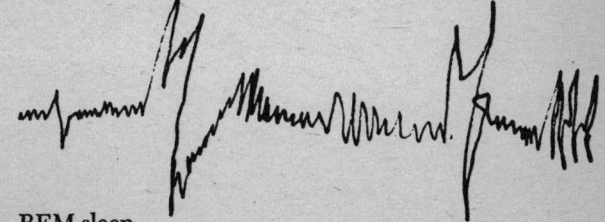

REM sleep

something, and you dream, this is the part of sleep we are all most curious about.

Why do we have a REM sleep? The evidence to prove the theory that REM sleep is caused by a chemical/physiological process was collected from cats. It was found that an electrical shock to a certain portion of a cat's brain will cause the feline to go into REM sleep. But if a cat has just gone through REM sleep and is shocked, the animal cannot be induced to reenter a REM period. This indicates that REM sleep is caused by a bodily process, and the amount of REM is controlled. Evidently a certain amount of REM is needed, and no more than that will be tolerated. Also, REM sleep must be followed by a period of NREM slumber.

Sleep is not a relaxed, resting time, it is a cyclic experience of unmoving brain activity as well as muscular movement. That is the normal sleep process. Yet some people, when they lie down at night, do not get a "good night's sleep." We'll look into this problem in the next chapter.

3

Dreaming

A dream is a fantasy—a mental process that is quite different from the way we think when we are conscious. The logical rules that govern our awake thoughts do not rule in the world of dreams. Real objects and situations, true relationships between individuals, and the world as it really is has no place within our dreams. Dreams are often fanciful, sometimes fearful, and they can reflect thoughts and feelings we had when we were much less mature than we are today as adults. Dreams are private experiences. Although dreams are true fantasies, they can seem as real to the dreamer as anything that has ever happened during the awake hours. During dreams there is no true fear of consequences; we can yell, condemn, love, or hate during a dream, and sometimes we even commit crimes.

It has been calculated that we spend approximately four years of our lifetimes dreaming. You readers who claim that you do not dream should realize after reading chapter two that you do dream, but you simply are not remembering your dreams. Different cultures look upon dreams from different perspectives. The Senoi tribe of Malaysia teach their children to dream in particular, specific patterns. Supposedly, these people also train themselves to eliminate nightmares and to add artistic thoughts to their dream patterns.

Throughout the history of man, people have tried to understand what dreams are. Perhaps the most persistent question that has been studied and argued is "What causes dreams?"

In the 1900s, scientists decided that it was possible to test theories about the causes of dreams in a scientific fashion. One experimenter tickled the noses of sleeping subjects with feathers, held burning matches close to their faces, dropped bits of water on their skin, and shone bright lights in front of their eyes. He concluded that as each stimulus was applied to the subject, a relevant dream resulted. Other researchers speculated upon the effect of the dreamer's own body in relationship to the content of the dream. Edgar Allen Poe's tale "The Telltale Heart," in which the sleeper confuses his own heartbeat with exterior sounds, is an example of this thinking. In other words, these scientific workers believed that the dream was the result of a specific stimulus and that there was a direct connection between the subject matter within the dream and that which was going on or had gone on during the subject's conscious life.

Freud believed that dreams were a natural protection for the sleeper to keep him from awakening prematurely. As an individual would begin to awaken and sleep would become lighter, dreaming would occur. This, he believed, prevented the individual from becoming completely aroused. This type of thinking was called the "guardian-of-sleep" theory. When REM sleep was discovered, the guardian-of-sleep theory persisted for a number of years. It was thought that REM periods of sleep occurred due to a full stomach, a nagging bladder, or the sound of a police siren.

This theory was extensively tested by researcher William Dement, whose results were quite unexpected by the guardian-of-sleep theorists. One of Dement's experiments involved the drinking of nearly a quart of water prior to going to bed. According to the guardian-of-sleep theory, these individuals should have REM periods as a way of handling their full-bladder thoughts. If the need to urinate affected the dreams of an individual, one would assume that the result would be REM sleep, dreaming, and then awakening to go to the bathroom. Yet Dement's subjects apparently did not dream of having to urinate. The results of these tests indicated that none of the results anticipated by guardian-of-sleep theorists occurred.

Dreams, then, are apparently not the result of internal or external stimuli. An external happening may be incorporated into a dream, but will not be the direct cause of the dreaming. For example, one researcher sprayed water on sleepers and then woke them to find out if their dreams incorporated a spray of cold water. One of the dreamers related his dream, which involved a leaky roof with water dripping down on one of the characters in the dream.

Sigmund Freud would have looked upon modern researchers' attempts at understanding dreams with chagrin. In his famous psychoanalytic book *The Interpretation of Dreams*, Freud told a story involving the wife of a policeman who had dreamed that her house had been broken into. She yelled for help, but the policeman nearby had walked up some steps and entered a church. Behind the church was a hill with woods covering it. As the policeman entered the church, the dreaming policeman's wife spotted two shabbily dressed individuals with aprons accompanying the policeman. Freud found this dream significant. Female genitalia were represented by the church and the steps were a symbol of sexual intercourse. The woods covering the hill were pubic hair and the hill itself was a Venus's mound. Freud believed that dreams contained the clues to a person's unconscious thoughts. All the wishes, fears, and instincts the patient might hold hidden within his or her mind would be revealed through the interpretation of dreams. Although some dreams might be difficult to analyze, there was a hidden meaning in all of them. Since people want to understand their dreams and the meanings surrounding them, Freud's theories became accepted and are still popular today.

Freud was not the first to believe that the true soul of an individual was apparent through the interpretation of a dream. Primitive Fijian islanders believed that the soul departed within a dream and the dream itself was a way to view one's own inner being. The ancient Egyptians—almost four thousand years ago—interpreted dreams much as Freud did in the early 1900s. The Greeks also used dreams as a way of understanding their lives and formed dream rites to heal sick individuals. The Iroquois Indians believed that dreams were commands and that if one dreamed of being told to do something specific that dream must be followed. Medieval Europeans were scared of their dreams; if devils and witches could enter their dreams it was then a quick trip into their bodies. Dreams were interpreted by the Inquisition judges; one was often burned at the stake as a result of dream interpretation. Ancient Jewish rabbis had a saying, "A dream that is not understood is like a letter that is not opened."

Throughout the ages, civilization has yearned to understand and interpret its dreams. Since Freud's time, psychiatrists, psychotherapists, and psychoanalysts spend a large portion of their time interpreting the dreams of their patients. If an Egyptian had dreamed of carrying his father's head on a plate, the family would have considered themselves warned of a foreboding incident. Freud would have said that the boy was expressing a castration wish. However, we have not found a satisfactory answer to what causes dreams within the subject matter of the dreams themselves. One thing we can see, however, is how dreams change our bodily functions.

Dreams are an every-night occurrence for all of us, usually about four or five times during the sleeping period. If the dream is a frightening one, the pulse quickens, the eyes dart around, temperatures change, and breathing becomes uneven and difficult. The body, however, remains limp. It is as if a storm has invaded the body, but its wild activity is not noticeable from the outside. It is fairly easy for the experimenter to enter the mind of the dreamer. The encephalograph indicates when REM sleep begins. Usually the subject is given about five minutes before being awakened by a buzzer. As the evening wears on, usually the buzzer will not be sufficient interruption to awaken the dreamer and repeated calling of his name might be necessary. The subject will find that every time he has awakened he has been dreaming. As the dreamer relives his dream, the experimenter is usually once again awed by the detail, color, smells, sounds, and sights that are included within the dream. Usually by the time morning arrives, the dreamer has forgotten most of his or her dreams. Since a normal individual dreams about every ninety minutes all night long, for a total of about one and a half hours of dreaming per night, an unbelievable amount of activity takes place within his mind. Yet if an individual is not sleeping in a sleep laboratory, he or she is usually unaware that all this activity has taken place.

Freud and other psychoanalytic theorists—each with their own individual viewpoints—believe basically that our psychosomatic illnesses and neuroses are intertwined with our dreams. As we repress and hold down basic drive impulses during the daytime conscious hours, these feelings and impressions manage to exhibit themselves during the night via dreams. They believe that a person's psychological well-being and the way he manages to handle his or her basic human drives are connected in a significant manner to her or his dream content. Since Freud's theories were first developed, REM sleep has been discovered. As scientists studied the REM cycle, they came to the conclusion that perhaps sleep was the result of the REM cycle, simply a side-product. The body when asleep still has a certain amount of excitation within it, and the visual and cortical centers of the brain continue to work during REM sleep. The only human materials that our biological systems have to work with while we are sleeping and not conscious are our feelings, thoughts, and memories. These are the makings of dreams.

Although dreams are probably the result of physical organization, this does not mean that our psychological needs are not being fulfilled during dream periods.

There is a biological and psychological mixing involved in REM dreaming. Although the cause of dreaming may be physiological, the content of dreams is nonetheless unique and magnificent, sometimes bizarre, often colorful, filled with imaginary thoughts, smells, and sensations—and this aspect of dreaming cannot be held up and analyzed with physical methods.

4

A Full Night of Sleep

What is a fine night's sleep to one may leave another feeling groggy and washed-out. Different individuals require different amounts of slumber a night.

There are always reports of people who do not need sleep at all; these have never been substantiated within the laboratory setting. It is true, though, that some require precious few hours of rest—and for them this is the best amount to have. Years ago, two Australian men claimed that they needed only an amazingly small three hours of sleep a night. When checked in a laboratory for a period of one week, it was found that they actually required a bit less than three hours of sleep. Yet they awoke fully rested. It should be pointed out that they were monitored twenty-four hours a day, and took absolutely no catnaps during other hours. They simply required far less sleep than the rest of the population. Some people consider themselves insomniacs because they require a low amount of sleep per night. If you awake feeling rested, and

A Full Night of Sleep

the feeling continues throughout the day, you are obviously getting all the sleep your particular body requires. Be pleased that you have many more waking hours within which to pursue life than do the rest of us unfortunates who sleep away about one-third of each day.

Sometimes one needs a certain amount of sleep over a period of years, and this sleep requirement changes —often quite suddenly. A Dr. Janesson slept about eight hours a night throughout his adult years. At forty-two he took a trip to Europe for six weeks, and when he returned to this country, he went to bed as he always had at eleven o'clock. Yet, instead of awakening at his usual seven in the morning, he found that he was awakening at three o'clock to three-thirty, night after night! He began to read in the middle of the night—he was a medical doctor and was always behind in his following of the literature pertaining to his specialty—and continues to do so until this day. He always awakens after four hours of sleep or so, and has about three or four hours of reading time while the rest of his family—and the world—sleeps. He is delighted with the set-up and does not in the least miss the hours of sleep that he used to experience prior to his trip.

There is really no known medical explanation for Dr. Janesson's case. Probably the fact that he took a trip right before the change is coincidental. Perhaps there was a hormonal change... we just don't know the answer.

The usual amount of sleep for a teenager is about ten or eleven hours; when he reaches college age, he requires less, and sleeps about eight hours. Often as people age, they require a bit less, but there is usually not a significant change in later years.

One exception to this is the case of pregnant women.

They definitely require more sleep than they did prior to pregnancy. The usual increase is about two hours a night (or day). This is probably connected to the profound hormonal changes which take place at that time.

It was thought at one time that babies needed huge amounts of sleep, say twenty hours or so in a twenty-four hour period. Those of you who have had young children know this is not so. In fact, researchers have proven that the average sleeping time for newborns is about sixteen hours in every twenty-four hours. And many infants sleep a great deal less and are quite normal and healthy. Some sleep as little as five hours, to the great consternation of their parents!

Salvador Dali has a unique way of napping which insures him a short amount of sleep but, he claims, sufficient rest. A metal dish is placed upon the floor next to his comfortable chair. He holds a spoon in his hand, and places his hand over the plate. He manages to hold on to the spoon until the exact moment of sleep—that is, when he can no longer be aware of his environment and cannot remember that he is supposed to be holding a spoon. At the moment that sleep overcomes him, the spoon drops onto the plate and the clattering awakens him. The artist says he feels just fine after this miniscule amount of sleep. He claims it refreshes him and recharges his batteries. This is amazing when one considers that the only sleep he has had is the time between the spoon's leaving his hand and hitting the dish! So much for sleep stories. . . .

The usual question asked of sleep experts is "How much sleep do I need?" The answer is that no one really knows if you need sleep at all, much the less how much! We only can calculate how much people, in fact, do sleep. And, of course, it seems clear that we *do* require sleep, since no one has ever been found who is healthy and does not sleep at all. I personally do not think we will ever find such a person.

One thing we do know is what happens to people if they are deprived of sleep. The classic experiment of sleep deprivation was done in 1894 by a French scientist. She took a group of puppies and did not allow them to sleep for about five days. They all died. They could not survive without slumber.

When a modern scientist repeated this experiment and then did an autopsy on the sleep-deprived animals after death, nothing was found to account for their death. They died of a lack of sleep, but it was not clear what part of the organism broke down under the strain and caused death.

Laboratory studies have shown that people who are not getting enough sleep react in a hostile way to others. In addition, they have trouble performing lengthy tasks. Prolonged procedures boggle their minds, although if the task can be completed within a short period of time they seem able to cope with it. Those of you who do not get enough sleep do not have to be told how it affects your whole being. It can truly ruin all the awake hours. But why do you not get a good night's rest?

Let us look first at the young child. In certain cultures, the youngster does not sleep alone and away from the parents as they do in our "civilized" environment. Also, in poorer homes the child often has a number of people sharing his room, and sometimes his bed. I would like to do a study someday to determine if these poverty-stricken people, when they grow into adults, have fewer insomnia problems than do the remainder of the population, for I believe that many problems relating to sleep start during the childhood and infancy years.

Often bedtime is an unpleasant time in many households. Sometimes a child is offered bribes to go to bed; the prodding goes on for hours in some homes. Dr. Spock's old advice to put a child in bed with love and affection, and then close the door no matter how loud the howling is and despite the fact that it might go on for hours, is not followed by many of American parents. This is understandable but unfortunate. The child should enjoy the bedtime hour; sleeping in a comfortable place when one is tired is an enjoyable experience. Yet many children have somehow gotten the message that going to bed is a punishment (perhaps it *is* used as that sometimes—"If you do not eat your food, I'll send you right to bed.") and they do not want to partake of the enjoyment.

One part of the trouble might be that the child has terrible dreams when asleep, and is afraid to fall asleep because they will recur. This is a sound complaint and one that parents must respond to. Usually a child has not yet mastered the vocabulary adequate to describe the horrors that he or she has experienced, and the parent will sometimes downplay the terror of it all. "Don't be silly . . . there are no such things as dragons." This sort of a response is definitely neither persuasive nor comforting. The parent, while explaining that there are, in fact, no existing dragons, must show sincere sympathy for the child's feelings and thoughts; they must indicate that Mother and Father understand how terrifying the whole thing is for the child. Assurance that they will always protect and care for the child is the correct tack to take. These scared children who sleep alone have formed poor sleep habits which plague them for the rest of their lives.

Bed is a large part of our lives. We are born in a bed and usually we die in a bed. As teenagers, we whisper secrets to friends at slumber parties right before we sleep, and as adults we have intimate relationships with others while in a bed. The bed has a great deal of meaning to all of us, and our feelings regarding it must overlap into our general sleep habits.

Perhaps if anthropologists stayed up at night and slept more during the day while studying various societies, they would have greater insight into the thoughts and feelings of the various peoples. Sleep customs—the way people prepare for it and what they do while in bed and as they sleep—are a key to many unknowns and are only recently being explored by scientists as deeply as are, for example, eating habits. These feelings about sleep are vital to the understanding of cultures.

The bed itself holds a place in people's feelings toward sleep. Did you know that there are very few people who can fall asleep if they try to sleep with their feet at the head of the bed? A fetish to be sure, but it certainly affects sleep patterns. Try it and see how it feels. Today's modern bed is luxurious. There are water beds, and huge, super-long, super-wide beds. Mr. and Mrs. Nelson Rockefeller once bought a bed which is a work of art as well; and there are now sheets available beginning to resemble works of art. Many consider the bed the *only* acceptable place for sexual intercourse. Sleep, the bed, and sex are intertwined to the point where some individuals cannot fall asleep without indulging in sexual activity. Marriage counselors are familiar with this complaint.

Although people in our society seem to be quite fussy about their sleeping arrangements, when there is a war or similar upheaval of normal routine, the need for sleep still exists. Then sleep takes place in filthy clothes, in foxholes, with bullets flying overhead. In horrible, painful situations, people still sleep.

During World War Two, people used to the ultimate in comfort while sleeping slept in unthinkable conditions at concentration camps—seven men sharing a plank of wood, nine feet long, with two blankets to protect them against the bitter cold and resting their heads upon their shoes, slept. Perhaps as they slept, they escaped. They dreamed of better days and, at least for a few hours, felt no pain.

Sleep *is* an escape. It has been found that, when someone knows that the coming day is going to be unpleasant, they tend to oversleep and are hard to awaken.

It is unnerving to think that although people can sleep in the most inconvenient situations yet when some individuals appear to do all they can to go to sleep, and are really tired, they nonetheless do not sleep.

It is obvious that personality traits and psychological differences are related to sleep problems. You must take what you have to work with—yourself and your problems—and mange to work it all into a situation where you'll be able to sleep well. It is difficult sometimes to decide if a nervous person does not sleep well or if the individual is high-strung because he or she is always tired and worn-out due to a lack of sleep.

5

Sleeping Styles

Perhaps the concept of a family unit first took hold as humans—who needed to sleep—stayed in groups for protection during slumber. As they slept, they were protected from what was probably a frightening dark period where danger lurked, unseen. These long hours of darkness would have been difficult to deal with if awake. Sleep relieved the caveman of his fright of the unknown and unseen. Sleep was comforting.

People sleep in all sorts of manners, and have an endless variety of rituals which they go through prior to lying down for the night. How you prepare for sleep affects the way you sleep, or the trouble you have *trying* to fall asleep. Changes in pre-sleep rituals can aid you in your quest for rest.

Do you say "I really have a hard time trying to get a good night's rest. I fall asleep easily but awaken after only five hours," as a patient of mine did recently? She was tall and tan from the sun and her twenty-seven-year-old face did not *show* the strain of lack of slumber. Her eyes were bright yet, as she talked they took on a worried look. "My husband falls asleep at about eleven o'clock; I usually try to go to sleep then also, but end up turning on the news and then watching Johnny Carson. This bothers my husband. Then I try to sleep again. After about an hour, I turn on the bedside light —which my husband tells me disturbs *his* sleep—and read for an hour or so until I feel sleepy ... finally! I end up sleeping very soundly for about five hours and feel rested when I awake, but I know I must be tired. I have to be with so little sleep. My husband is worried about me and suggested I come to see you."

It was clear to me that this young woman's only problem was her own and her husband's thinking on sleep patterns. Although her mate required about eight or nine hours of sleep, my patient did not. Yet because he was in the habit of going to sleep at an hour which would allow him his optimum amount of sleep, she was trying to mimic him with her body. It was not working.

I explained to the attractive young woman that she was not an insomniac at all. She then asked if I could give her a pill so that she could extend her sleep period to the same length as her husband's! "Are you sure there is nothing you can do so that I'll sleep a normal eight hours?" After further discussion, she was finally convinced that she was sleeping a perfectly normal five hours, and should continue to do so. She did not need medication. We worked out a solution to her problem. She set her under-the-pillow alarm to wake her up hours before her husband awoke. In this way she slowly changed her going-to-bed time to coincide with her husband's, and got up early enough to do all her household chores prior to having breakfast with her husband and leaving for work. She continued to be well-rested, and her husband was satisfied with the solution, for his wife bedded down with him. He was not disturbed when she awoke early in the morning as he slept on.

Another patient told me that his family went to bed at nine o'clock every night and expected him to do so also. He would lie in bed for hours prior to being overtaken with sleep. He usually fell asleep finally at about twelve o'clock, after three hours of trying. We placed this patient in the sleep laboratory. The result was that the indicators of natural awake-periods and sleep-periods in an individual—heart beat and body temperature—remained fast and high until about midnight which indicated that his body was not ready for sleep until that time. His family's and his try at fitting his body into a mode that the rest of the family followed was simply not going to work. After explanations with the patient's family, the boy was allowed to go to sleep at midnight and all of his insomnia-related problems were solved. In fact, they never did actually exist. From then on, the patient crawled into bed at the proper time for him and fell asleep instantly.

Let me re-emphasize that *there is no number of hours of sleep which we all need.* It varies with the individual. What is good for your mate might be all wrong for you. Look at the Questionnaire you filled out at the beginning of this book with an eye toward spotting the sort of problem these two patients had. Are you sleeping a specific number of hours nightly, night after night? Are you going to bed several hours earlier than appears to be necessary? Are you sure you really have a problem? Or are you convinced of this because other members of your household simply require more sleep than you do? Your "need" for sleep is established by your body, not by some medical text or your next-door neighbor. And so is the amount of sleep children and babies, and elderly people, require. Do not assume that an individual, because he might be very old or young, needs more or less sleep than you do. It might not be so.

The statistics on the number of hours various people sleep within a twenty-four hour period are interesting. A scholarly article that appeared in the *Journal of Medical Science* in 1962 revealed that eight percent of the individuals studied slept a very small number of hours nightly, five hours being the cut-off figure. There were included in this eight-percent group several who slept less than this. About fifteen percent slept about five or six hours, and the majority—sixty-three percent —were in bed sleeping from seven to eight hours a night. One group, thirteen percent of the total people studied, required more than eight hours of sleep, sleeping from nine to ten hours a night. There were even a few—two percent—who needed more than ten hours of slumber daily. It is clear from this study that the commonly-held theory that we all need eight hours of sleep a night is false, and has no basis in fact. Extract that old-wives tale from your mind.

We mentioned earlier that infants have as varied needs for sleep as do grown-ups. It stands to follow that a newborn requiring huge amounts of rest will, as he or she grows into a toddler, a teenager, and finally an adult, continue to need larger amounts of sleep than the one who never needed much sleep at all.

Parents brought their five-year-old into my office one day. They had made the rounds of many specialists and were weary from their search for someone who could help them. The problem was that the child did not sleep enough. No matter what time he was put to bed, he slept only about five hours. Although he looked healthy, the mother and father knew he could not be. What could they do for their poor, sleep-starved child?

As we talked, the parents were prompted to remember that the boy had *never* slept very much. Even in the hospital nursery everyone had commented on how "wide awake" he looked compared to the other sleeping figures. As an infant, he was up all night and, amazingly, all day too!

I explained that their child needed less sleep than they did—which they had some trouble accepting—and would grow up to be one of those people with the benefit of several more productive awake hours than the general population had access to. After our discussion, they accepted their child's rather unusual sleep requirements, and there was no longer any problem. Of course, there actually had never been any difficulty. If the parents had thought back in time, they would have realized that their child had required little sleep from the day he was born. This should have given them a clue about his present sleep patterns. Just as you would not purchase a pair of shoes for your child that were the average size for a person of that age, do not expect yourself or your child to sleep an "average" amount of hours.

If there is anyone who is envious of persons who require little sleep, like the young boy just described, it is the scientists who study them and find out this fact! A colleague of mine was up at two o'clock one night staring at a chart of a sleeping subject who claimed he only needed three hours of sleep a night. He had fallen asleep at eleven. The sleep scientist was particularly tired that night, for he had been up the night before with another volunteer and had spent a good part of the day "working up" the data the instruments hooked up to the previous evening's subject had fed out to him. He himself had gotten in only a catnap of three hours of sleep in the late afternoon. So he was actually beginning to doze off when his subject suddenly awoke, jumped out of bed, and looked as fresh as a daisy! My researcher-friend was so angry; if there is anyone who would like the facility of requiring a small amount of sleep, it is the sleep researcher! This particular one crawled into the subject's vacated bed and slept soundly until morning.

Just as there are many different amounts of sleep required by various individuals, there are also many different ways of getting that required amount of sleep. Some people sleep in pajamas and some do not. Some people like to sleep in underwear. Individuals may sleep uncovered, with only a sheet, or with goose-down blankets—and all of them may be sleeping in the same climate. Some have windows open, some have the room sealed. Big, soft pillows are available, yet certain people like hard foam and others prefer nothing at all. There are all shapes and types of beds and some sleepers move around a great deal in them. There are people who roam *all over* their beds while sleeping. Some awake with their feet where their heads started. Some jitter while sleeping ... they look as if they are dancing and playing the piano at the same time. Some people wear terrible expressions on their faces while they sleep, others look perfectly peaceful. Some people sleep with a foot or a hand in the air; others sit up and stand up—and even walk—during their resting hours. I once studied a man who looked as if he were lifting weights as he slept. His arms kept going up and down. When awakened, he said he was dreaming of giving his baby a bottle! Heads, arms, and legs can either move almost constantly or never move, depending on the individual. And all of this is quite normal and does not seem to affect the quality of the sleep. People do different things during their waking hours, yet when they show individuality as they sleep, others think they need medical help. This is not so.

A study was once done to try to determine if certain types—psychological and physical—slept in somewhat the same manner. The researcher thought he did detect such a trend. He first described three types of humans, based mainly upon their physical characteristics:

Endomorph— heavy, fat individuals who are soft and flabby; these people delight in eating a good meal.

Mesomorph— muscular people, often large-boned; enjoy exercise.

Ectomorph— skinny, fragile, sensitive people; nervous, apprehensive, pipe-thin arms and legs, alert.

While these are very generalized slots to place people in, the researcher who did the work did see the following patterns relating to the specific types:

Endomorphs love sleep, enjoy it thoroughly... they sleep soundly... usually snore... can sleep in any situation and position... are completely relaxed... might be termed "gluttons" for sleep ... extremely hard to awaken.

> *Mesomorphs* do not particularly care for sleep, consider it a waste of time ... like to be awake and doing things ... require little sleep, often as little as six hours ... loaded with energy ... no problem going to sleep but is very active while asleep, twisting, turning, wiggling ... snores loudly ... cannot recall dreams.
>
> *Ectomorphs* are insomniacs ... do not sleep regularly, and did not as children ... every little sound awakens them ... find it hard to crawl out of bed in the morning ... light sleepers, do not really relax even when asleep ... dream ... feel tired even after a decent night's sleep ... do not usually snore.

While these classifications are extremely simplified —almost to a fault—they do show some tendencies that are valid. The part that inheritance plays in the quality of sleep an individual experiences might be great, if one believes that the basic personality traits are at least in part inherited.

Often a run of night-owls will show up in several generations of one family. People describe themselves as "night people" or "day people." There is a physical explanation for this: the body temperature. There is a normal "high" and "low" in an individual's body temperature daily. When it is low, a person feels worn out and tired. At the high peak, there is a lilt to one's walk, and the person feels like conquering the world, or at least the dinner dishes. Some people show a higher rise within the time of one day than do others; others hit very low lows. People who wake up and jump out of bed with " a song in their hearts" usually will show a rapid rise to their daily high; folks who are active in the evening hours can have as high a high, but their body temperatures rise more slowly, over a longer period of time. This all could have a connection with an individual's genes. Variants in body-temperature highs are sure to cause trouble within a family at one time or another. However, these variations must be accepted because body temperature is a function of our body's built-in regulating system, and we cannot change that.

You must not judge yourself—insofar as sleep is concerned—in comparison with others. You are you. This is something every insomniac must come to terms with. Your own particular sleep is related to your body and your personality as well as your heredity. Really, the only way to decide if something is wrong with the way you sleep, assuming there is no medical abnormality that might have been present for many years or a lifetime, is to consider how you slept prior to realizing you had a problem. Do not decide something is wrong because Joe sleeps more soundly than do you, or Jane sleeps twice as many hours. If there is a change in what was always normal for you, then worry and concern are warranted.

Sleep is a part of your total make-up, and includes connections with the way you spend your awake hours. It cannot be separated from the complete picture of you. If you do not awake refreshed as do many others, if you feel as if you have been fighting all night and wake feeling like a sodden mass of matter sure that you have not really slept at all, try and accept it. For one thing, it is extremely hard to estimate how long we have slept, and how "well" or "soundly." One of the reasons for the Sleep Questionnaire was to enable you to better gauge what is really happening to you at night. Try to look at yourself realistically. Do you really have a problem, or are you making one for yourself where one does not exist?

6

You Are a Clock!

In the last chapter, we mentioned that mechanisms within your body have an important effect on your life and can affect your whole being, sleep in particular. The mechanism that is most profoundly related to sleep is what is sometimes called the "clocks of life." These are the systems within you which regulate the very tempo by which you live, and die. These biological clocks cannot be tampered with. Yet as modern society forces changes upon us, our internal timing systems suffer.

For example, when one takes a jet trip through time zones, morning is turned into nighttime and fatigue and general tiredness are the result. We cannot tell our internal clocks to reset themselves. For instance, it takes several days for our bodies to get back in synchronization with our surroundings after a time-zone change. As scientists see the results of this modern jet travel, they begin to reconsider an old question: Do we really need sleep, and must that sleep be at night? Why do we sleep at night rather than, say, in the afternoon?

Long ago, as was mentioned in chapter four, sleep was a form of protection. It seemed safer to huddle together and sleep than to wander around in the night. But also, of course, one could not hunt in the dark. There was nothing to be done in the night except rest. However, today this is no longer true. Consider the possibility of half of the population sleeping in the daytime and working at night—with the aid of electricity—while the other half rests at night as usual. One-half of the world's population—and a great deal of crowding, especially within cities—would disappear from the streets. Fewer cars would crowd the roads at any one time. The schools could be used to top efficiency. But how would it affect our total beings?

Almost everyone seems to sleep for an extended period every twenty-four hours. The usual amount of this sleep is five to nine hours. Although it has been rumored that there are cultures that do not work this way and, in fact, that certain societies take several short naps rather than having one protracted sleep period, researchers have not yet found concrete evidence of any such societies for confirmation of these tales. So we will assume that, whether it is habit or necessity, most of the world sleeps generally as we do in America. There are cultures, such as in South America, where an afternoon nap is regularly taken. But these people still sleep at night for the major part of their resting period. In areas where there are months of darkness, again people do much as we do. A Norwegian study was done which indicated that the people there sleep an average of seven hours within a twenty-four-hour period during the summer months when there is daylight at "night," and about eight hours in winter, when it is dark day *and* night.

Our bodies seem to be geared for a twenty-four-hour day, with the one period of sleep within it. There are billions of components within us that need to be controlled by some centralized timing mechanism or the body simply would not work. Virtually all forms of life have to have some sort of controlling device such as this. Plants move their leaves according to their internal clocks, also on a twenty-four-hour basis. If one moves a plant to a dark cave, the same regular motions will be made by the leaves. Lobsters and fishes have a resting period. Even clams slow down; their respiration becomes slower for a certain period of time every twenty-four hours. Although insects do not have the same sort of resting period as humans, the famous nineteenth-century naturalist Julian Huxley described what ants do in their form of rest:

> They may choose a depression in the soil as a bed, and there lay themselves down, with the legs drawn close to the body. When waking (after some three hours' rest) they behave in a way startlingly like that of our proud human selves. The head and then the six legs are stretched to their fullest extent, and then often shaken; the jaws are stretched open in a way remarkably reminiscent of our own yawn.

If you have an aquarium, sneak up at night and turn on the light. You might find that some of the fish are actually resting on their sides at the bottom. Toads and frogs also have a resting time when they are very quiet and still; and, of course, birds sleep.

You Are a Clock!

The tides are part of our timing system of twenty-four hours. They come in and go out, controlled by gravity from the moon, on a twenty-five-hour basis. Certain fish lay their eggs in the spring on beaches. They somehow—their clocks within them—know when the high tide occurs and lay their eggs immediately following its peak. This gives the eggs the best chance of surviving before the next high tide occurs, for low tide follows high, and it takes about thirty days for the next monthly high tide to occur.

If you were to take an animal that reacts in a certain way to the tides away from the ocean, it would still continue to follow tidal activity. For instance, mollusks—which do not have brains—react with nerve impulses to tidal changes. When they are placed in an aquarium within a laboratory thousands of miles from the ocean, they continue to respond to the far-away tides via their inner clocks; their nerves still "feel" the tide and react to it. No one is sure quite how.

Prior to civilization's understanding of internal biological clocks, people throughout the world sensed the connection between the moon, the tides, and inner clocks. They planted and harvested according to tides and full moons; they knew that reproduction was somehow connected to all this and developed fertility rites around them. The menstrual cycle, approximately every twenty-eight days is an example of our clock at work and its relationship to the lunar calendar. The fish laying their eggs just following a high tide are an indicator of the connection between reproduction and the moon as the moon controls those tides. Ancient peoples recognized these correlations, and developed religions around these observations.

Scientists who first studied the biological clocks

within all organisms wished to find out if they were indeed internal. Were animals responding to something inside, or were they simply noticing the position of the sun, or the amount of light or darkness? A study was done with bees that answers these questions. Bees in France were trained to come to a particular spot for feeding at a certain time every day. These same bees were then flown to the United States, where the time differs. If the bees watched to see how high the sun was in the heavens to aid them in getting to their feeding spot on time, they would arrive at nine o'clock in the morning, just as they did in France. But if, in fact, there was something within them which told them when to go to get fed, they would arrive at the feeding station (which also had been transported to the United States) at what was nine o'clock in France, but a different time, clock-wise, in the United States. The bees, following their inner clocks, arrived at the feeding stations exactly twenty-four hours after their last feeding in France, so that it was not yet daylight in the United States while it was light at nine in the morning in Paris. Within three weeks, however, they had adjusted to the new time and were finally eating at the same time, clock-wise, as they had in France. Man makes this same sort of an adjustment as he gets over what is commonly called "jet-lag," after flying through time zones.

Although many animals are not light-lovers, as are we humans, we all are kept on schedules internally. Bats, owls, and cats seem to be more alert at nighttime than in the day. In the case of the cat, scientists have established an explanation. The cat's eye—which perceives the darkness—sends a signal to that part of the brain that controls sleep and arousal. When lights are switched off in a laboratory, the signal immediately sent to the brain of the cat can be measured on instruments. It tells the cat to "come alive," to be alert. If this mechanism is surgically removed from the cat, the feline begins to act like a dog at night. That is, it is no longer overly alert in the darkness, and goes to sleep.

Humans, on the other hand, seem to be exactly opposite to the cat. We awaken and become alert with the light. However, scientists have not as yet located the mechanism that controls this in humans and are uncertain if it works in exactly the same manner as the cat's.

This rhythm that controls our lives to such a great extent is called *circadian rhythm*, from the Latin words *circa dias*, or "about a day." That Latin term describes our internal rhythm pattern or as we revolve within a twenty-four-hour day. This inner timing can affect us if we are operated upon in a hospital—our chances of recovery depend upon the resting period of our whole systems—and all our activities throughout the day are connected to this timer. The way we think and feel, our ups and downs—our inner clockworks have a lot to say in all of this. And, of course, our sleep is affected.

One measurable effect of our body clocks is body temperature. Throughout the twenty-four-hour cycle, our temperature changes about two degrees. This temperature fluctuation is constant and reliable; it rises in the daytime and falls in the evening. It usually is at its lowest in the middle of the night, between two and four o'clock. The average human feels fine when his body temperature is high, and will be in horrible condition if he or she happens to be awake when it is at its lowest. Workers who are employed at night have been studied and it has been found that, at the low point of their daily temperature scale, they feel miserable, physically. They develop chills, and feel dirty and sloppy. Many accidents occur during this period. Words become slurred, and judgment falters. This is especially evident in such people as stewardesses, pilots, doctors, and factory workers, who have been on the night shift for years. You have probably seen this sort of a reaction in yourself.

The circadian rhythm is strongly within us. As trips in space were planned, medical scientists wondered what would happen if men were taken away from gravity, sunlight, clocks, and the social goings-on that guide their lives, such as bedtime. They had some information to base their speculations upon.

In 1938, Nathaniel Kleitman and a companion entered a cave that contained an underground cool cavern. There they arranged living quarters and remained for over a month. The purpose of this expedition was to test the theory of environmental effect upon the human being in relationship to his circadian rhythm. They tried to change their usual schedule. They set up an electrical connection, and in the absolute darkness of the cave they were able to change night into day by turning on the light. And at any time of the day, they could turn off the bulb and they simulate nighttime. They first tried a schedule which was based upon a twenty-one-hour day. This worked. They ate and slept according to this cycle and were able to adapt. Then they attempted to live a long day of twenty-eight hours. This was much harder. The younger companion managed finally to adjust, but Kleitman, who was in his forties, could not. No matter what he did, his body followed its lifetime pattern of

You Are a Clock!

twenty-four hours, seven times a week. To live the longer day, he had to have a six-day week. He found he was awake when he most needed and craved sleep, and was having trouble trying to sleep during what his body thought was daytime. He was testing a bit of futuristic jet-lag.

One group of people which is profoundly affected as was Kleitman by the need to stay within one's own body's clock is commercial airlines pilots. The fogginess experienced when one is working at the wrong time in one's personal rhythm can be literally killing for the pilot and his passengers. Airline company physicians have noted premature aging in pilots; the fatigue and constant time-zone changes are difficult on their systems. Overseas stewardesses experience an uncommon amount of menstrual irregularities. This fatigue suffered by night workers and people who change their exterior rhythm due to time-zone changes is not simply a feeling of tiredness.

A cave explorer lived 390 feet within the earth. Although when he emerged he thought it was mid-August when it actually was mid-September, while he was in the cave in total darkness, his body—without the help of a man-made clock—had adhered to its circadian rhythm and continued to react on the basis of a twenty-four hour day. His clock—and the one within you—is extremely accurate and reliable. We must pay it heed. For to do otherwise affects our whole being, and, in the end, the clock wins the battle one hundred percent of the time anyway.

7

What Affects Sleep?

Age. The main influence upon your sleep is age, that old bugaboo. It is well known that the elderly have more sleeping problems than do the rest of the population. As we discussed previously, sleep habits change with age, sometimes sensationally. The way you sleep at age twenty will not be the way you do so at sixty, and what is a normal night's sleep for you as an older person would not have been right for you as a teenager. The main difference will probably be that the sleep of the older being will not be as deep and satisfying as it was earlier in life. If you are in your later years and consider yourself an insomniac because you cannot recapture the way you used to sleep years ago, you have misdiagnosed yourself. You are simply getting older. This message is for those of you in your forties and fifties, also. You'll never again have the high quality of sleep you experienced years ago. This change can be caused by many factors. Probably it is the result of a metabolic slowdown, hormonal differences, and a decline in energy and muscular strength.

Numerous studies have been done on thousands of people and their sleep habits. They have revealed that the older a person is, the more chance there is that she or he will complain of poor sleep patterns. The seventy-year-olds complained of insomnia seven times as often as did the twenty-year-olds.

Actually, there is not such a great difference between young adults and their older counterparts in total number of hours slept. It is more the quality of the sleep that differs. The unbroken, sound sleep of the younger person is a thing of the past for the oldster. Sometimes a partial reason for this is more catnapping during the day. As a person ages, he has more freedom and it becomes possible, as it was in infancy, to take a nap whenever he wishes. These people often do not count this day-sleep toward the full amount of sleep that they have within a twenty-four-hour period. In fact, studies have shown that often elderly people who think they are getting less sleep are, when the day-time naps are counted, sleeping more than they used to! However, an older person must actually lie in bed longer than a younger being to collect the same number of sleeping hours, because the aged individual takes longer to fall asleep and awakens more frequently during the night. It has been calculated that a person in his sixties spends about sixteen percent of his time in bed awake.

People find that as they age it is easier to wake up and become alert after slumber. This is because the type of sleep that the older person partakes in is less deep; there is a smaller amount of NREM Stage Four sleep during the night. Also, an older person spends less time in REM sleep which, as you remember from chapter two, are the times of dreams and rapid eye movements. An infant, on the other hand, spends about fifty percent of its sleeping hours in REM periods. During the learning years, REM sleep still makes up a sizable chunk of the sleeping hours. In the older person, it declines. It is interesting to note that, although elderly people experience less time in REM sleep, they are better able to recall dreams than their younger counterparts. This could be because they have, over the years, taught themselves methods to aid them in remembering dreams. Or it could simply be that they awaken more frequently during REM dream episodes.

The number of complaints I hear from the elderly concerning sleep problems makes me wonder if they really are sleeping as little and as poorly as they suppose. Perhaps the older person with sore joints might awaken him or herself when turning over while asleep during the night, whereas a younger person would probably just turn over and stay asleep. Also, older people are more prone to coughing after lying down for a period of time, and perhaps this disturbs their slumber for a minute.

Catnaps. I think also I must bring up the familiar scene of an aged relative before a fire, dozing and snoring aloud, who is indignant when someone mentions that he or she has been sleeping. "I have not! What are you talking about?" The elderly seem not to be able to recognize their smaller episodes of sleep as well as they did when they were younger, or they refuse to accept them as part of the aging process.

There is no question that our senior citizens are reluctant to own up to the fact that they have been dozing when they are caught at it. They also hate to admit to their doctors that they take a nap during the day. Yet this sleep-time must be considered as a part of the total amount of sleep a person gets.

Sex. Unlike catnaps, patients do not mind placing the blame for their sleep problems on sex, however. Sex has always been associated with bed and sleeping. A private, quiet, dark place where it is comfortable to disrobe—this description fits bedtime as well as a sexual encounter. Many people have the notion that they are insomniacs because they crave sex and, without fulfillment, they cannot get a decent night's sleep. But is this really so?

The concept that one sleeps after sexual intercourse is deep-grained in our particular society. This is partly because sexual activities usually take place prior to bedtime, so it is logical to then fall asleep. But the fact is that most people could engage in strenuous activity within three or four minutes after sex and would feel invigorated as they exercised. While it is true that the orgasm is a relaxant to the muscles, there is no basis in fact that this is the *only* way to feel relaxed enough to be able to manage to fall asleep at night. People who feel that sex is a necessary prerequisite for sleep and are insomniac without it, have a psychological, not physical, problem. That is, they have talked themselves into thinking something which they wish to believe. Studies have proven over and over again that sex is not a necessary act prior to healthy, restful sleep. The connection is only in the mind of the beholder.

Habitual Bedmate. The habit of sleeping in a double bed with a particular mate is another story. Studies have proven that when one is used to sleeping with a certain individual the absence of that partner from the bed will cause a disruption in the lone person's sleep

patterns. This particular research was conducted on young medical students who had been married at least one year, but not more than three years. Evidently the anxiety of sleeping alone caused a reduction in REM sleep, thus disturbing the subject's full night of rest.
Gender. Sex differences also play a part in the overall patterns of sleep. According to recent surveys, there are approximately two female insomniacs for every male. This statistic must be softened with the word that women are more prone to discuss their medical problems, and the true figures would probably not show such a pronounced difference between the sexes. There is evidence that women age more quickly than men do insofar as changes in sleep patterns are concerned. Women tend to fall into the problematic habits of old-age sleepers at an earlier age. Men seem to show variants in their lifelong slumber habits at about age sixty-five; women start to change their sleep patterns at about fifty-five.

The most common sleep problem that women encounter is sleepiness during pregnancy. There are females who can tell when they are pregnant prior to the cessation of their periods by the overpowering desire to sleep. Usually this desire for sleep becomes less pronounced after the first few months of pregnancy, but not always. During pregnancy, women sleep soundly and feel rested when they arise, which is often in contrast with their usual, nonpregnant habits. The action of hormones plays the major part in this change.

Drink. Chemicals ingested as drink also affect the sleeper. The drink most often associated with insomnia is coffee, and there is a valid reason for blaming the beverage for the sufferings of many insomniacs. Of course, the solution for these people is simple: They can simply not indulge in caffeine prior to bedtime. However, it should be remembered that coffee is not the only caffeine-containing beverage; tea and cola also contain the chemical. A twelve-ounce bottle of cola contains approximately two-thirds the amount of caffeine found in one cup of coffee. There are many arguments about the effects of caffeine on different individuals. There are people who have a cup to help them fall asleep, and they swear it works! And certain individuals can drink cup after cup all day long and have no trouble sleeping. Others have one cup and truly cannot sleep. It seems to me that the individual who drinks a lot of caffeine regularly is not as affected by it as the person who only has a cup once a week. It is much like the effect of alcohol. A nondrinker is going to react more readily to a scotch and water than will the individual who has one every evening. Again, if caffeine is your problem, you do not have to read my book to know that you have the solution available: Simply do not indulge.

Coffee—containing caffeine—is a stimulant so it makes sense that it might keep some people awake. Alcohol, on the other hand, is a depressant and puts certain people to sleep. Yet alcohol—like coffee—does seem to have a reverse reaction at times. People can grow nervous, irritable, or high when ingesting alcoholic beverages.

An excessive amount of alcohol seems to reduce the amount of REM time during sleep at first; later the REM sleep catches up and most of the night—too much—is made up of REM sleep. The individual who has a drink prior to bed to help himself relax and sleep might eventually be fooling around with the natural sleep processes, causing himself to awaken in the middle of the night during a bad dream. If you rely on nightcaps to help you sleep, make sure the quantities stay small enough to only make you a bit drowsy. Otherwise, although you might sleep a full night's number of hours, you will not be getting the right *kind* of sleep and will awaken feeling tired and "hung over."

Exercise. A commonly held belief is that exercise helps one sleep. Yet too much exercise can be stressful and have the opposite effect. If you wish to use exercise as a "sleeping pill," make sure you do it regularly and do not overdo it. You need not be exhausted to benefit from exercise. Usually if you are overtired from exercise, you will have more trouble sleeping than if you had not exercised at all. Exercise in moderation.

Comfort and Cleanliness. People of certain cultures will not go to bed unless they are absolutely clean. Showers and baths are extremely relaxing, as are clean sheets and bedclothes. You should make sure you are as physically comfortable as possible as you prepare for bed.

Atmosphere and Environment. You must do everything you can to create the right setting for yourself in particular as you set about to go to sleep, for the insomniac is much like the fabled princess who felt a pea beneath ten mattresses. If you have trouble sleeping, every little thing adds to the problem. Your bed companion might be "sleeping like a log" while you thrash around in a room that is too hot, even though you just got out of bed and turned up the heat because you had decided you could not sleep because you were cold. A bark of a neighbor's dog wakes you; the mattress seems to have lumps in it. . . . Read on; I'll help you.

8

Insomnia—Man's Universal Malady

The true insomniac lives in hell. All day long, as he drags his tired body around in a sluggish manner, he wonders, "Will I get any sleep tonight?" Most patients who enter my office have seen many doctors about their problem over a period of years. They have taken prescription medications and tried old-wives'-tale remedies, and still cannot sleep. The first thing that must be ascertained is whether or not there is a medical problem lurking beneath the obvious dilemma.

I once had a patient who complained of insomnia and stated that he had not had a restful night's sleep in the past thirty years. He looked twenty years older than he actually was, and did indeed appear supremely tired. Absolutely nothing helped him. After testing in a sleep laboratory, we found that the gentleman was suffering from one of the most terrible illnesses associated with insomnia: *sleep apnea*. Sleep apnea is detected with the aid of instrumentation, for sufferers of sleep apnea, unbelievably, cannot breathe when they are asleep.

This man would fall asleep for about ninety seconds. One could see from the machine measuring respiration that he was *not breathing at all* during that time. Suddenly, the man would awake, take several gasping breaths of air, and fall asleep again, only to awaken in another minute and a half to give his air-starved lungs another bit of air. This is the way this person slept; it was no wonder that he felt tired all day, every day.

The interesting thing about sleep apnea sufferers is that they usually complain to their physicians of sleeping *too* much. These people find themselves falling asleep at all hours and in many circumstances during the day. It is certainly understandable when one considers how many times they awaken in the course of one night's sleep. Their central nervous systems, which control breathing, shut down when they fall asleep, stopping the muscles which facilitate breathing from working. At the same time, the throat muscles collapse. The body undergoes a profound shock, which awakens the sleeper, who then gasps for air.

There are some sufferers of sleep apnea who are not aware that they have the malady. They apparently immediately fall back to sleep after each episode so that it does not overly affect their overall sleep benefits. There is a theory that some people are born with this problem and that perhaps crib deaths may be related to it. At present, the only treatment which seems to help is the surgical insertion of a tube through the throat into the airway. This disease is not well known among physicians; although millions of patients complain of sleep problems, the medical professions really are in the Dark Ages as far as knowledge and medical treatment of these sleep disorders is concerned.

Insomnia—Man's Universal Malady

Another sleep problem that profoundly affects the lives of the sufferers is *narcolepsy*. A woman is driving a car when someone behind her suddenly beeps his horn. The woman collapses onto the steering wheel like a mound of Jell-O. This woman has the disease that causes a person to become essentially paralyzed when there is a sudden, unexpected sound or when he becomes highly excited. For example, if this same woman were to start to laugh, she would collapse to the ground with a bounce as she hit the floor.

Narcoleptic individuals also suffer from drowsiness during the day, occurring rather suddenly and causing havoc with their lives. But it is the severe episodes which cause them to drop to the ground that make the leading of a normal life impossible. People suffering from this disease have reported that it is impossible for them to spank their children when they are angry—the emotion makes them collapse. A gunshot will cause them to slump to the ground. The sudden movement of a bird in flight caused one sufferer to fall and break a collarbone.

Most of the day the sufferer is an average individual, alert and aware of his surroundings. But at times a wave of sleepiness overcomes the narcoleptic rather suddenly and he can do nothing to prevent it. In some instances, the patient will fall asleep almost without knowing it. There is a report of a patient who fell asleep while scuba diving at forty feet under the ocean! Another physical and social problem for these people is that sleep frequently overtakes them during the sex act.

The sufferer of narcolepsy—when falling asleep at a sudden sound or because of a strong emotion—is falling into REM sleep, often while right in the middle of performing an activity. In REM, or rapid-eye-movement sleep, vivid dreams take place yet the dreamer stays asleep because of a sort of paralysis that enables the sleeper to continue to sleep while dreaming exciting and frightening thoughts. The inhibitor that stops the normal sleeper/dreamer from hopping out of bed during a dream is mistakenly put into action at the wrong time for the narcoleptic. It suddenly inhibits while he is awake, not sleeping. It makes him fall down and actually be asleep, instantaneously.

This disease, which shows up in certain family lines, usually begins between the tenth and twentieth years. Although this is probably the first time you have heard this disease described, it is not rare. Probably about a hundred thousand Americans suffer from it.

We *have* all heard of *sleep-walkers*, *bed-wetters*, and *sufferers of nightmares*. These problems usually occur in young children and often disturb the parents more than the youngster. These are NREM disturbances and may have more of a connection with physical situations than most people recognize. For example, bed-wetting may often be caused by a weaker-than-average bladder which, during relaxed slumber, tends to lack the control it would have in the daytime. These sorts of problems also run in families, and most children outgrow them prior to adolescence; they should probably NOT be treated unless there is valid indication of a physical problem. Patience is really the only cure. Save your money, parents, and wait it out.

It is extremely important to ascertain exactly how many hours you do sleep. It is common—about fifty percent of my patients do this—for a person to think that he or she is not getting enough sleep when in fact the individual is sleeping a full night of slumber. The only positive way to find how many hours of sleep you are getting is to enter a sleep laboratory; these are few and far between. Perhaps your mate can help you to analyze carefully your total sleeping time. Study your Sleep Questionnaire and search for areas you are not sure about. See if you can obtain the true facts in some manner. Even if you feel tired and groggy during the day and you are sure you have not "slept a wink," your finding out that you did in fact sleep many hours *must* have a psychological effect on you. You might be feeling exhausted because the type of sleep you have is close to being awake and does not fully rest your body. Or your feeling of lethargy could be caused by some medical problem.

A patient came to me recently with little hope and a lot of despair. She was miserable. I listened to her complaints and found that she was getting as little as two hours of sleep a night, according to her reckoning. She was truly unhappy. Yet careful studies indicated that she was actually sleeping nine hours every night, at least for the week we tested her! The experience of this patient points out that complaints and descriptions of horrible insomnia have little or nothing to do with the actual amount of sleep a patient is getting! This particular patient, who for years had tried everything from warm drinks to sleeping pills, was considering retiring from her job as a stock broker because her chronic insomnia was leaving her so "washed out" that she could hardly think during the day.

When this patient was informed that she was sleeping a sufficient number of hours during the night, she was greatly surprised. Usually patients with the identical complaints this woman had are given sleeping pills. This is the worst thing that could be done; she *is* sleeping, and the medication will only cause her in the long run to sleep *less*.

I could not tell this patient *why* she felt that she was

not sleeping. Her exhaustion during the day was real, and obvious to me. Her condition, called *pseudo-insomnia*, is impossible to diagnose without careful records of sleep patterns, for a doctor has no way of knowing whether a patient just thinks he is not sleeping, or whether he really is *not* getting the needed rest.

With this patient, the knowledge that she was getting a large number of hours of sleep relieved her. The possibility of her continuing with a regime of sleeping pills for the rest of her life was quashed. A month after I diagnosed her, she visited my office again. She looked better rested, and generally healthier. She said to me "My worrying over my loss of sleep has stopped now that I know I am indeed sleeping and getting a good night's rest. I find that I am not waking up as often as I used to in the middle of the night and so do not feel as unhappy and depressed as I did before coming to see you. Generally I am less tired."

Many insomniacs sleep nine hours a night, while people who feel rested and happy with their sleep might sleep only about five hours. Insomnia is not clearly understood by the medical profession. Research, although only taking place in a few laboratories throughout the country, is searching out the mysteries of insomnia.

There are many faces to insomnia. The next four chapters will discuss more fully pseudo-insomnia, or imaginary insomnia, as well as situational insomnia and emotional insomnia and voluntary insomnia. Continue to refer to your Sleep Questionnaire as you read through these chapters, and see if you fit into any of the descriptions of sleep problems.

9

Imaginary or Pseudo-Insomnia

Many years ago a patient of mine was also my next-door neighbor. One day he complained to me, as he had many times in the past, that although he had actually spent a full seven hours in bed the previous night, he had not slept one minute of that long, drawn-out block of time. The conversation changed to other things and after several other topics of conversation passed between us, I asked him what he had thought of the robbery. "What robbery?" he asked. I then described the hoopla that had taken place at the house across the street from our homes the night before, with police cars, flashing lights, spotlights, sirens, the apprehension of the thieves, and all the accompanying details. Both my friend and I suddenly realized that he had slept right through the whole thing! Unfortunately, only one of us admitted that fact. He kept insisting that he had been up and alert all the night through. Considering what went on during the night, there was no way an awake individual could have missed it. It had *awakened* me, my wife, and my children.

Marriage counselors know that people are often not aware when they are awake and when asleep. Many a wife has complained of a husband's snoring while the husband, furious, has stated that he had never even been asleep. His anger is partly based upon the fact that the following day he *feels* sleepy, and knows that he cannot have slept because he is physically miserable. It infuriates him that his wife can be so unsympathetic. This sort of a scene can go on to the point where it disrupts marriages.

This problem and that of my next-door neighbor become more understandable when people such as these are wired to instruments and studied. The results indicate that they are often close to the line between wakefulness and sleep, in a state of suspension, not really awake or sleeping. Their nights are filled with episodes of light sleep, bordering on actually being awake.

This problem of deciding whether one is awake or asleep is not only a problem with the uneducated or ignorant. I remember the first time I was a "subject" in a sleep laboratory. The room and the bed were strange; the wires attached to me were cumbersome. I twisted and turned all the night; when I finally crawled out of bed in the morning, I wondered if I would be able to face the many patients I had to see that day. I apologized to the monitoring scientists; I had not been a very good subject—they had probably obtained very little "sleep" data from me. They looked at each other and laughed. Then they showed me the vast amount of information they had obtained while I slept—for a full seven hours, one-half hour longer than I usually sleep at home! From that moment on, I sympathized with and better understood the complaints of my "imaginary" insomniac patients. It is almost impossible to ascertain the amount of sleep you actually have in a given night. The state of wakefulness that hovers just under the sleep act is hard to differentiate from wakefulness itself. If you feel you have not had a decent night's sleep for weeks or months, consider the possibility that you are, in fact, getting a goodly number of hours of sleep, but you are not sleeping as deeply as you would wish. You think you are not sleeping—but you are.

There *are* people who have been asleep and do not believe it. And there are other individuals who are told by others that they have been awake and they themselves are quite sure that they have been sleeping! These people sleep with their eyes wide open. It sounds rather uncomfortable and "unnatural," but it is so. The Chinese have an old legend surrounding the phenomenon of sleeping with eyes open. In the third century A.D., a general ordered three tailors to sew three thousand outfits in a period of three days. This, of course, was impossible, yet the general ordered that it be done on time or the tailors would be assassinated. The tailors collectively decided that they must murder the general to save their own skins. Late at night they crept into his bedchamber. They were about to stab him when one of them noticed that his eyes were open and he was looking right at them. They fled. Later they listened outside his door and heard snoring. They entered the room, again ready to kill. The general was still staring at them, yet he continued to snore! They killed him.

The explanation of this tale, which has been marveled over for centuries, is that the general was one of those people who regularly slept with his eyes open. Studies have been made on these people wherein objects are held before their open, sleeping eyes. The subjects are then awakened and asked what they were thinking. Their thoughts during slumber had no connection with the object which had been placed within seeing distance of their open eyes. When a sleeping person sleeps with his eyes open, that individual is, during the sleeping period, blind. This is true no matter how lightly the person is sleeping. He cannot see the object, even if he insists that sleep did not overtake him and that he was in fact awake. He was unseeing.

Let us go back to the problem of the imaginary or pseudo-insomniac. Why is it that these people are so sure that they are not sleeping? Although they appear to be complainers and to remember only the time they do not sleep, which in some cases is only minutes a night, the fact is that the sleep that they are getting is somewhat different from the sleep experienced by those who do not complain of insomnia.

Look at the case of a thirty-six-year-old male who complained of life-long insomnia. When tested in the sleep laboratory, we found that he did not take very long to actually fall asleep and then proceeded to sleep about eighty-five percent of the time he was in bed, or six and one-half hours. The quality of his sleep was fine also. He had a goodly amount of REM sleep and enough of the four NREM stages to feel well-rested. But he did not. Why?

The changes from one level of sleep to another are usually regular and smooth, as indicated by measurements of brain waves. Yet this man's travels from one level of sleep to another were erratic and uneven. Some of the cycles were not completed; he did not ride the crest of a regular, smooth night's rest, which is a rhythmic up and down. He went up a bit then down for a while. Then he would shoot up for a while, and suddenly down again.

We tend to regard all sleep as a restful, quiet way of recharging our batteries. But this man's style of sleep clearly showed us that there are different kinds of sleep, and some are not as restful and fulfilling as are others. As certain people's sleep differs from the norm in that it is less smooth, their pulse-beat rates and heart temperatures are higher. Maybe these poor sleepers have a different rhythm from the rest of us, and are forced into the style of living they follow by society. Their body temperatures do not rise and fall in the same manner as the average person's does.

These people appear to me to be psychologically and physiologically unique. There is data to suggest that insomnia and emotional illness are intertwined in some way. One good way of diagnosing approaching mental deterioration is to study sleep patterns. Of course the lack of sleep—and satisfying rest—does affect the mental outlook of these sorry sufferers.

Another difference between the insomniac and the sleeper is in the dream department. Insomniacs remember dreams better; they know when they have awakened and, when an experimenter awakens them, they often claim to have been awake prior to being formally awakened. They are lighter sleepers. They remember a great deal of their thought processes from their sleep periods. Probably the reason they think it takes them longer to fall asleep initially than it really does is because they remember their thoughts in their early moments of sleep, so they think they are awake during that period. Probably the same thing happens prior to their awakening.

Let me state clearly that imaginary insomnia is a

serious matter. These people are not getting the sleep they need, and it is not easy for them to understand exactly what is happening in terms of their sleep needs.

Nothing could be more irritating than to have people laughingly tell you you have been asleep when you not only *know* and *feel* that you have not, but are exhausted from the "lack" of proper sleep. Imaginary insomniacs do not feel asleep when they are. Perhaps their bodies are not resting as others do; maybe they are in a heightened physiological state during sleep. Their bodies might be, in actuality, awake although their brains are not, according to instrumentation analyses.

It is hard to pigeon-hole the imaginary insomniac; the best way of course is via the sleep laboratory. But if you find people refuting the fact that you have been awake when you *know* you have been, consider the possibility that you are a sufferer of imaginary insomnia.

10

Situational Insomnia

Every human being has, at one time or another, suffered from situational insomnia, which is often caused by a crisis. The businessman who has a big deal pending will be tense and unable to sleep. I had a patient once—a hardworking plumber—who had bet two weeks of his earnings at the horse races and had lost his money. His tense feelings were as real to him and as strong as the general who would be planning to attack in the morning. Emotionally upset or worried people cannot sleep well. The odd thing is that they expect to be able to sleep just as they did before they were upset.

Several years ago, a well-known, very successful businessman came to my office. He had been suffering from insomnia for over a year and had tried all sorts of cures. None were successful. Every night, he was unable to sleep in the middle of the night, for about two hours. He had gotten into the habit of reading in these small hours of the night, but he wanted to sleep then.

After an hour of conversation we found that the reason for his insomnia was an episode that had taken place over a year ago. A business deal involving half a million dollars had been negotiated by this man over a period of four months. The project had been very frustrating to the gentleman, and everything that he did, both socially and in business, was affected by this crisis in his life for a time. Unfortunately, the business deal did not go through, and he was angry, upset, and frustrated. Although this episode had taken place quite some time ago, he still felt anger as he recalled the incident. He did not realize until we sat and discussed it how much this aborted business deal was still affecting him.

After our conversation and several other conversations the businessman had with a psychiatrist, he began to sleep better. The built-up anger within him had caused a prolonged case of situational insomnia. This patient's particular problem was obvious both to him and to his doctor after a short period of conversation, but others often have much more deeply hidden reasons for their insomnia problems.

One patient of mine, an attractive, intelligent young woman, came to me for help because she was unable to sleep, although she had never had a problem sleeping before in her life. This particular episode of insomnia had lasted for six months prior to her coming to me for help. I could not help her, although I did spot signs of situational insomnia within her, so I suggested she see a psychiatrist.

After two visits the psychiatrist discovered the reason for her insomnia. Her husband was having an affair, and this deeply hurt and angered her. She had said nothing to her husband—he was unaware that she knew of his extramarital activity—and she had not spoken of it to friends or relatives. Her emotional turmoil was surfacing in her sleep problems.

As I said previously, we have all suffered from this sort of insomnia at one time or another in our lives. We have all felt dejected, we have felt helpless at one time or another in our lives, we have been angry and upset with situations within our daily lives, we have been tense, lonely, and unhappy.

Sometimes we are unable to sleep because of simple changes within our daily routines. One gentleman who was used to sleeping a full eight hours a night found that he was unable to sleep when his wife and two daughters went on a trip for a month, leaving him alone with two dogs and a goldfish. He could not understand his problem. His daily occupation included exercise, and he felt tired at night. He was not upset, although he did miss his family. When his family returned home once again, his insomnia disappeared.

Adults are not the only ones to suffer from situational insomnia. An exam can keep a teenager awake, and we all know what the anticipation of Christmas does to younger children. My own child had a period of insomnia when he was about six years old. My wife and I began to think that perhaps he was emotionally disturbed, for we could think of no reason to cause his problem. This was during a period of time when I was working very late at the office and would usually come home after my young boy had gone to bed. After several conversations I learned the reasons for his sleeping difficulty. He was trying to wait up for me! I altered my schedule so I could be home to eat dinner with my young son and his problem disappeared.

We do not have separate minds and bodies for our

awake hours and our sleeping times. That which affects our emotions when we are awake will also make an impression upon our sleeping hours. It is strange, in fact, that people complain about not sleeping well when they are upset by something. It would seem obvious that our sleep would be affected by emotional tension and strain. Our emotions are not separate from our body chemistry. Our whole being is affected by our mental outlook to the point where various chemical reactions take place within our systems when we are angry, upset, frightened, or lonesome.

Scientists studying sleep via the sleep laboratory actually cause patients to suffer situational insomnia. When an individual offers to be a "guinea pig" in a sleep laboratory, that person soon finds himself or herself wired up to several different instruments with a tiny thermometer in the rectum. As their pulse, temperature, respiration and brain-wave patterns are measured, scientists find that these people suffer from what they have termed "the first-night effect." The volunteers feel somewhat uneasy and anxious during the first night in the sleep laboratory; they do not sleep as they normally would at home in the bed that they are used to, surrounded by their familiar personal things. During "the first-night effect" the subjects often skip their first REM sleep period. Other abnormalities in their sleep patterns are evident also. Often it takes several nights of sleeping in the sleep laboratory for the subjects to start sleeping in whatever their usual, normal pattern is. Of course, not all subjects will react in the same way to the anxiety and stress that is present within the sleep laboratory set-up.

Just as people react in an individual manner toward stress in the sleep laboratory, individuals going about their daily activities show a variance in the way they react to life situations. We all know people who get tremendously overwrought from the smallest disagreement with another person. On the other hand, there are people who don't seem to be bothered at all when they have heated, loud, boisterous arguments with others. Also, not everyone will react to stress and strain with an onset of situational insomnia. Usually, however, stress, tension, and anxiety, if severe, will affect sleep. Serious matters such as the loss of a job, the break-up of a marriage, or the death of a loved one, will upset an individual enough to cause the onset of situational insomnia. The uprooting of one's family also causes stress and strain in certain individuals.

In 1963 a study on the uprooting of families was conducted by Norman Bradburn, a psychologist from the University of Chicago. A large company in Sioux City, Iowa, was transferring over a thousand of their workers to another part of the country. The company was concerned because in the past whenever a transfer was necessary, many workers decided to quit rather than to go along to the company's new location. They were interested enough in this phenomenon to agree to let Bradburn conduct a study during this period. The Chicago scientist considered sleep patterns a significant factor in analyzing the overall effects of stress upon individuals.

First, the individuals involved in this study were asked if they had had sleeping problems prior to the announcement of the plan to transfer. Interviews followed over a period of several weeks, and the same question was asked again and again, "How are you sleeping?" The result of this study was that although some of the people were having trouble sleeping, and others felt a bit more nervous and a bit less energetic, generally the incidence of insomnia among these people was really only slightly higher than would be found among the general population. These workers were under stress, but it was not affecting them to the point that it was causing severe insomnia.

Bradburn's findings are not so surprising if you look at situations around the world. A person's background and culture have an effect upon what sort of experiences will cause him to lose sleep. For example, during World War Two the people of London suffered incessant, mind-boggling air raids. Many of the Londoners had a great deal of trouble sleeping. The bombing went on for almost two years. There were individuals who never had a decent night's sleep throughout that long period of time. Yet, as people gathered together in the bomb shelters there were always those souls who slept as if they were in their own beds with no stress or strain surrounding them. And, of course, the ability to sleep during stress situations is not indicative of the English people exclusively.

The Balinese culture acts in a rather unusual way—at least from a Westerner's point of view—when there is danger, trauma, stress, or tension. Let me quote Margaret Mead's observations of these people:

> If you were to come home during the middle of the afternoon and find all the servants asleep, you would know that something was wrong—they had broken something.

These people go to sleep whenever there is trouble! If a woman is giving birth to a child she will not, as individuals of other cultures would, have her children

Situational Insomnia

removed from the area, because when she does, in fact, begin to deliver and even prior to that while she is in labor her children, feeling somewhat tense and knowing that something unusual is happening, will lie down and go to sleep. If a Balinese gets into serious trouble, he goes to sleep. A thief will fall asleep during his trial. Nobody at this point has studied the dreams of the Balinese people; I feel it would be a very interesting research project.

The evidence of the Balinese would seem to indicate that we react to stress and strain in the manner that we do not because it is instinctive, but as a cultural habit. The Balinese react to the same sorts of stimuli in a completely opposite way than most Westerners do. This is obviously a learned behavior pattern.

However, although most Westerners will react to problems, agitation, and trouble with nervousness and will generally find it hard to sleep when such feelings occur, there are some people in our culture who do react to problems with sleep. We call these people *hypersomniacs*. I have a number of patients who do complain of suffering from the opposite of insomnia—that is, too much sleep. These people also have difficulty awakening and it takes them what they consider to be a protracted amount of time to be completely alert after a slumber period. There are people who, when there are difficulties within their lives, find that they sleep a great many more hours than usual, sometimes up to twenty hours a night. Yet when they awaken in the morning they do not feel well-rested and refreshed. Perhaps these people, like our ancestors the cavemen and women, are sleeping to escape their problems. There are people who are doing psychoanalysis and will fall asleep right in the middle of the session rather than discuss their personal feelings, problems, and anxieties.

Some people suffering from hypersomnia do not realize it. They do not connect over-sleeping with their feeling listless and unrested, but assume that the reason they feel that way is some other medical or emotional problem. They do not even consider the fact that their sleep might not have been truly restful for them. This is understandable after such a sleep—it *is* hard to believe that one could not feel rested after sleeping a huge block of time.

At the same time, a number of individuals blame insomnia for difficulties that have nothing whatever to do with their lack of sleep. Of course, insomnia can magnify other problems because the resulting exhaustion affects everything that an individual does throughout the day. I sometimes have a patient come into my office who seems to be overly worried about his or her lack of sleep. Some patients will complain about a lack of sleep for a period as short as one week. This sort of a problem does not really warrant a visit to a medical doctor who is a specialist in sleep problems. I believe that these individuals come to me because the hours that they would usually spend sleeping are by now becoming additional time to worry, feel sad, and generally suffer psychic pain. These patients sometimes decide their insomnia is *the* great hardship and problem of their daily lives.

Some individuals suffering from psychological problems zero in on insomnia as the basic illness to be treated. There is a danger in this deception. Doctors will often go along with this analysis of an individual's problems and prescribe sleeping drugs. This, as you will find in chapter thirteen on drugs and medication for sleep problems, is only compounding the original difficulty. Such people are deceiving themselves, and self-deception of this sort can be very injurious to their mental and physical health. The treatment usually ascribed to insomniacs will do these people absolutely no good, and will only divert attention from the actual root of the problem.

These same people will go around talking to friends and relatives, acquaintances and doctors about their serious sleep problems. It is often easier to discuss insomnia than it is an unhappy marriage, disillusionment with one's job, problems relating to children, or money difficulties. Most physicians, unfortunately, will go along with the patient and accept the fact that the serious problem is his lack of sleep. They don't delve any deeper and do not recognize the fact that the root of the problem is unhappiness created by outside situations, and that the complaint of lack of sleep is simply a cover-up. It is also easier for a physician to treat insomnia—usually with drugs—than to try and help the patient with, for example, a marital crisis. When a physician will delve deeper into the problem and help the patient face the true reason for his insomnia, the problem with sleep often disappears.

A fine example of this sort of rationalization is a patient I am very fond of. Mrs. Sims had not been in my office for over two years. When she did walk in, I noticed that she had gained approximately a hundred pounds since I had last seen her. She complained of insomnia. This had never been a problem before in her life. She told me that she would awaken during the night almost every night. Since she had nothing else to do she would get out of bed, go to the kitchen, and have a midnight snack. As this continued to happen every night she began to put on a great deal of weight. Due to this weight gain she was forcing herself to stick to a strict diet all day long to make up for her overeating during the nighttime. This began to affect her whole outlook on life and her personality, and she began to lose her temper and yell at her young children rather regularly. Her husband was upset with this abrupt change in her personality. Mrs. Sims blamed it all on insomnia—if only she could sleep at night she wouldn't eat so much, she wouldn't have to diet during the day, and she would not be so grouchy. It never entered her mind that the fact that her mother was dying of cancer in a far-away city might be causing the insomnia in the first place. Mrs. Sims's problem was resolved in a rather unfortunate manner—her mother finally passed away, and Mrs. Sims started sleeping throughout the night. Her weight returned to normal and I have not seen her in my office since.

The death of a loved one caused another patient of mine to develop insomnia. Mr. Dolonik had a life-long friend who was killed in an automobile accident. Shortly thereafter Mr. Dolonik began to have trouble sleeping at night. Every time he would start to fall asleep an almost overpowering wave of fright would possess him. He felt as if he were going to die if he went to sleep. One time as his eyes closed, he imagined that the bedroom walls were going to crush him. Another time he was sure he was going to smother in his pillow. A couple of sessions with a therapist cured Mr. Dolonik of his mental anxiety due to the death of his friend. Coincidentally his insomnia difficulties ceased.

Mr. Dolonik's problem is a type that psychologists, psychiatrists, therapists, and social workers encounter often. The treatment for such problems is talk. Once these people understand that the basis for their insomnia is stress, tension, and apprehension, they can more realistically deal with their emotional upsets and they are no longer hidden beneath the trauma of insomnia.

Let me reemphasize that the treatment that most physicians normally suggest for sleep problems such as those articulated as situational insomnia, are in fact harmful to the patients—*i.e.*, drugs. It is so much easier for the physician with patients stacked in the waiting room to prescribe a sleeping medication than to listen to what the actual problem is. One must keep in mind that the average doctor has about five minutes in which to treat a patient who comes in complaining, for example, of a lack of appetite, a feeling of tiredness and insomnia. It is so easy to immediately zero in on the insomnia and prescribe what the physician considers to be the necessary medication. And, of course, this sort of treatment *will* help for a while, but only for a short time. The cause of the problem has not really been looked at and will crop up again within a matter of days or weeks. The drug route is harmful for a number of reasons, and this hiding of what the actual situation is can only be destructive for the patient. When insomnia is caused by crises in one's life, the only way to cure it is to recognize what the problems are and face and resolve them. In the case where there is no possible resolution of the difficulties, a clear, level-headed analysis of the problem can be helpful.

We seem to be looking at insomnia as if it were the plague. However, there are times where insomnia can be a helpful addition to an individual's life. When children are put to bed they do not worry about insomnia. In fact, it is rare for a child to have any sort of a problem that they will articulate in conjunction with falling asleep. Lying awake in bed is not considered, necessarily, a negative activity by the young. If the child is put to bed too early, it will usually spend the time in some way that is constructive for that particular child. We have all heard young children singing in bed, reciting nursery rhymes, and just talking to themselves. Many children spend up to half an hour talking to stuffed animals that they sleep with, discussing the day's events with a blanket, or admonishing a pillow for being naughty at lunchtime.

Teenagers also will lie in bed awake considering the day's events and often fantasizing. The hours in bed for children and young adults are often the only time of the day when they can feel as if they are completely alone with no disturbances or intrusions on their personal thoughts—a time of complete privacy. Although individual teenagers may sometimes dwell on problems when lying awake in bed, they often spend many moments or hours delving into pleasant times in the past, daydreaming, and anticipating future happy events. Pleasurable, fulfilling, happy dreams can be developed while lying in a quiet bed in the soft darkness of the night.

On the other hand, when adults cannot sleep, they generally consider themselves to have a serious problem. Rather than think about delightful situations their minds often wander over and over the problem of being awake instead of being asleep. They often worry about not getting enough sleep; there is the thought that if they don't fall asleep immediately the next day will be difficult to get through because of tired bones and groggy minds. Generally speaking, the more someone worries about being able to fall asleep, the harder, indeed, it will be for them to "drop off."

Situational Insomnia

We all have to deal with insomnia at one time or another during our lives. What we do during that period of time when we cannot sleep tells a great deal about our personalities and outlooks on life. People who get tremendously upset when they cannot sleep for short periods of time often are unhappy with their lives generally. Individuals who purchase sleep-aids of all sorts and who constantly go to their doctors to get drugs—and I am speaking of people who do not really have a serious insomnia problem—are overemphasizing their troubles with sleep. If they would spend as much time thinking of pleasant hobbies and outside interests that they enjoy, love of family, or other generally content feelings, they would find that their sleep problems would probably rapidly disappear.

My advice to people who are having trouble sleeping is to utilize their time in a constructive manner. It seems to me that it is a waste of time just to lie in bed and get upset. One could get out of bed and do some work, with the end result being a satisfying feeling of accomplishment. The middle of the night is also an excellent time to read. Many people like to try and write poetry in the darkness and quiet of the night. The middle of the night is a good time to do something that you have always wanted to do all your life but could never find time to. I recommended to one woman after a bit of discussion about things that she never has time to do that she revise her recipe collection in the middle of the night. For several weeks she sat and redid her index cards, went through a huge pile of recipes she had clipped out over the years from magazines and newspapers, and set up a file system so she could find various recipes when she wished to. Incidentally, as she started to engage in this activity during the middle of the night she found that her insomniac periods were slowly becoming shorter and shorter. The work—which she did sitting on her bed—seemed to induce her to sleep more rapidly than lying in bed counting backward, breathing deeply, or thinking of lambs jumping over a fence.

Not everyone feels like sitting up, turning on lights, and doing some sort of active chore. For those who want to lie in bed and rest, radio or television are excellent soothing time-killers.

It is silly to lie in bed and worry about not being able to sleep. It certainly does not help you fall back to sleep, and usually it will cause more anxiety, which of course increases your problem. If your problem is of a short-lived variety—that is, if you have had insomnia before but it usually only lasts for a couple of weeks or so—try not to get too upset about it. It will go away. No point in lying there and worrying about it. I am not referring to persistent problems with insomnia. A serious case of insomnia might indicate a serious medical or emotional problem that should be looked in to. You, however, must be the one to differentiate between the transient case and the serious, prolonged episode of insomnia.

11

Emotional Insomnia

The way you sleep is as distinctive as your thumbprint and your handwriting. If your handwriting were suddenly to change, you might suspect that there was some alteration in your personality. The same is true of your sleep patterns. When you are ill you sleep differently from when you are well. You have your own personal sleep patterns and these alter with bodily changes. For this reason sleep is an excellent indicator of emotional or psychological illness. Some day sleep recordings will be used in the diagnosis of mental illness as well as other diseases not related to emotional problems such as heart disease.

The most common cause of emotional insomnia is depression. There are many different levels of depression; we have all suffered from it at one time or another. Its symptoms range from mild "blues" and a sad feeling, to deep, dark gloominess, apathy, limpness, unhappiness, and heavy, unmovable melancholy. Some people swing between these different levels of depression on up to happiness and elation.

As depression takes possession of a person, sleep is affected, the personality begins to change. A famous neurotic, Oscar Levant, once described himself:

> During the most desperate phases of my mental depression which lasted many years, my most unabated obsession was constant unconsciousness.... A psychiatrist diagnosed my trouble as an abdication of will. I wake up and the feeling of terror is so knife-edged ... just the idea of waking up and facing the day of inertia and fear makes me long for a return to the unconscious.

Depression is a very common illness. Most often it affects the middle-aged. There are many types of depression, and the sleep patterns that depressed people display are varied. The usual complaint is that the person who is in a depressed state does not get enough sleep, or when he does sleep, does not feel rested when he awakens. In addition, he complains of the quality of his sleep. The sleep might be poor, fragmentary, unpleasant, or restless. It is unrefreshing. Another common problem is that these people seem to awaken quite early in the morning; this list of complaints is commonly known as diagnostic clues to depression.

While sometimes it is difficult to recognize that depression is the source of the trouble, certainly a complaint of insomnia is an excellent early-warning signal of emotional problems. Patients who often refuse to discuss that which is depressing them, or their depressive feelings, will discuss insomnia more readily. Unfortunately, as discussed in the previous chapter, they will often state that the only thing that is bothering them is insomnia and will not discuss anything else at all. They regard sleep as *the* major problem, and will not recognize the fact that the depression is affecting their whole being including their sleep patterns. These people feel that if only they could get a good night's rest, all other feelings of unhappiness or depression would disappear.

One kind of depression familiar to therapists is commonly called "smiling depression." An example of this was Miss Peacock, a forty-seven-year-old woman, unmarried, who lived at home with her elderly father, sister, and brother-in-law. She had an insomnia problem which presented itself at about four o'clock every morning. She woke up and could not sleep any longer, no matter what time she had gone to bed the night before. She belonged to several clubs and women's activities in the small town in which she lived and was always friendly and smiling, yet her family members knew that she was often depressed, unhappy, and bleak, and that these periods of depression overcame her quite frequently. One day her sister went down to the cellar to do the family laundry and found Miss Peacock hanging from one of the rafters. She had committed suicide. After her death her family looked back and realized that she had had disturbed sleeping patterns for a number of years and had been awakening very early in the morning for the past five years at least. They could not determine any particular reason or event which brought on her original insomniac problem and depression.

Often insomnia and depression are the result of a specific event, however. For example, another patient of mine, Mr. George, came to me very depressed and having a great deal of trouble with his sleep. Six months previously he had had a benign tumor removed from his neck. This medical episode had convinced him, however, that he was going to have a recurrence of the problem, develop cancer, and die an early death. After this episode he lost his appetite, was unhappy, and, although he had always been a shy, quiet-spoken gentleman, now he truly crawled within himself and became introverted and deeply depressed.

The particular sleep patterns of this gentleman indicated abnormal slumber. His patterns are rather typical of the depressed individual. He didn't sleep deeply and when he did sleep, it was for very short periods of time; even within these rather brief episodes of sleep he frequently awoke. His brain waves indicated that he experienced very little REM sleep or deep rest. He took quite a while to fall asleep and his sleep was generally erratic all night long. Mr. George's sleep—which did not include a normal amount of NREM Stage Four rest—was very unsatisfying to him. Normal people spend about twenty percent of their night within Stage Four sleep; Mr. George averaged about five percent. This was not enough for him to feel well-rested and bright and alert in the morning.

Although Mr. George experienced too little REM sleep, other depressed individuals engage in an overabundance of REM sleep. The point is that the sleep is, for that particular individual, irregular and generally erratic. If all sufferers of depression could enter a sleep laboratory prior to their emotional illness, and their doctors had at their disposal records of what would be for these particular individuals normal sleep patterns (measured by instrumentation), it would be quite obvious from patterns taken after the depression had set in that these people were sleeping quite differently than they had been prior to their emotional disorders.

Another sleep problem found in depressed people is dream-interruption insomnia. The normal sleeper does not awaken during a REM dream and then plunge directly into a second REM period, as happens with a dream-interruption insomniac. This sort of sleep would be confusing to the most normal, well-adjusted individual. A patient once described the experience to me thus:

> I keep waking up during the night thinking that I'm choking to death. Last night this happened about eight times. I absolutely cannot catch my breath. I realize that I am dreaming a few minutes after I have awakened, but when I first wake up it is frighteningly real. The strange thing is I cannot remember at all what my dream was about. This choking sensation has gotten so bad that I hate to go to sleep at night.

Researchers have determined that people who suffer from frightening nightmares are perhaps bringing on dream-interruption insomnia to awaken themselves from the horrifying dreams that they consistently experience. Their awakening numerous times during the night is a way to prevent dreaming, because their dreams are so horrible. The solution to this problem is to give these people a drug—carefully chosen—that will stop their awakenings but will not suppress their REM sleep.

Another sleep problem that affects depressed people is awakening in the early hours of the morning. A study was done several years ago in which a researcher made all sorts of loud, clanging noises while his subjects slept.

He had a group of depressed, emotionally unstable subjects as well as a group of normal individuals. He found a huge difference in their reactions to the noise he made during their sleeping periods. The normal group was essentially insensitive to the sounds he was making, particularly during their deepest periods of sleep. The emotionally unstable group of individuals, however, kept switching to a lighter stage of sleep when the noise was sounded. These people experienced less deep sleep to begin with than did the normal patients. They indicated an extreme sensitivity to their surroundings and environment during their sleep. I suppose that as dawn approaches and the sky lightens and more noises are heard out on the street, these people are awakened. This particular group was given anti-depressant drugs in the treatment of their illness and sleep patterns were again analyzed. It was found that their sleep was deeper and they were much harder to disturb with noises after the ingestion of anti-depressant drugs.

The non-depressed, "normal," healthy individual's sleep can be compared to the travels of a train on a circular track. The sleeper, like the train, travels along the track, stops at specific stations or intervals, starts up again, stops at another station, on a regular, clocked basis. In a normal individual, this round-the-track scheduled sleep pattern takes about ninety minutes. Depressed people do not show an orderly, circular type of sleep process such as this. Their stops are short and irregular. Their general cycles are fractured. The rhythm is all off and they do not have a normal night's sleep. Of course, there are other insomniacs who should not be classified as depressed, who also sleep in an irregular pattern such as this. Just as anti-depressant drugs will help the depressed individual who has an erratic sleep pattern, these same medications will often help the individual who is not depressed yet is sleeping in an irregular pattern and is insomniac. These particular types of drugs seem to reset the natural rhythm that determines one's sleep pattern.

We have discussed several types of sleep which are abnormal. But how can one tell whether one's sleep problems are simply insomnia, or whether they are actually pathological? Some of the answers to this problem can be found in the Sleep Questionnaire you filled out at the beginning of this book. The answers to these questions should indicate to you whether you should seek help with your problem. First you must compare the type of sleep you are having now to the type of sleep you used to have. Is there a difference? Is it heavier? Lighter? Or do you awaken more than you used to? Do you have nightmares now when you did not previously experience them? Any sort of change that is dramatic and persists could be an indication that you should seek professional medical attention for your problem.

Another question you should ask yourself is how long you have been having this problem with insomnia. Does it occur once a week? Every night? Once a month? Or several times within a period of a week? This is something that you should perhaps keep a record of. You might find that you are not having as much of an insomnia-type problem as you thought you were. On the other hand, the record might indicate that your problem is severe and occurs quite often. As you keep a record, try to indicate when you are having stressful daytime situations to handle. Along with your sleep problems, are you fatigued? Do you feel lethargic? Do you have trouble concentrating? Does your memory fail you often? Are you poorly coordinated? Are you irritable? Do you have trouble keeping your attention on a single matter?

Perhaps the problem that you are encountering concerning your sleep is of your own making. Study the next chapter on voluntary insomnia and decide.

12

Voluntary Insomnia—
The World Is a Marathon

For years, medical doctors have urged their patients who complained of insomnia to keep regular hours and do things in an organized, systematic way. In the past, there really was no factual evidence that this sort of treatment would be helpful for insomniacs, but today we do know that disorder in one's life and erratic living affect sleep. Our society is based upon efficiency, motivation, and attentiveness. We move quickly, and rest and sleep usually do not fit into our busy schedules. It is even hard to rest in a hospital. One is awakened early in the morning to have one's temperature taken and not allowed to sleep through meals or bathtime; a patient's sleep is constantly interrupted while in the hospital. My patients have often told me that they want to go home so they can get some rest!

Perhaps you are one of those individuals who set yourself up for bouts of insomnia. Do you ever cut your sleep short because you have to get up to take care of your many affairs? Do you postpone bedtime when you are busy with other things? Do you allow yourself to take a nap during the day when you need it? By cutting off only an hour or two of sleep a day you are affecting your whole being.

An interesting study was done by some sleep scientists in California. Volunteers were starved of sleep for several days and then were allowed to sleep a full night of restorative sleep. The day after their full night's rest they were given performance tests to complete. The findings indicated that even after a good night's sleep these individuals performed poorly. They were suffering the aftereffects of a lack of necessary sleep. Remember the puppies we mentioned some chapters back who, after being starved of sleep, died. There is a theory that after you have starved yourself of sleep because of a busy schedule or by getting up to feed a young child a bottle in the middle of the night for several months you may have permanently affected your sleep patterns. While this has not been proven positively, there is a possibility that a period of sleep loss could affect your future nights' rest. The aftereffects of fooling around with your sleep are evident when one studies a group of doctors. After a number of years of medical school and long hours of day and night working in hospitals, it was found that these individuals had poor sleep habits. They could not sleep at night. This insomnious pattern still manifested itself years after they graduated from medical school and were no longer having to cope with impossible nighttime schedules. This would seem to indicate that one pays for erratic schedules, possibly even for years.

There are individuals who consider insomnia to be an indication of their strong, forceful, hardworking personality traits. They almost feel as if they will not be considered to be highly motivated, hard-working individuals unless they complain of trouble sleeping. Hyperactive people often cause their insomnia themselves. High-powered, driven people do indeed have trouble lying down and relaxing for a long night's rest. If you have this type of a personality, you must force yourself to relax during the day and try to clear your head of occupation- or project-related details prior to your bedtime. You *must* make time for rest.

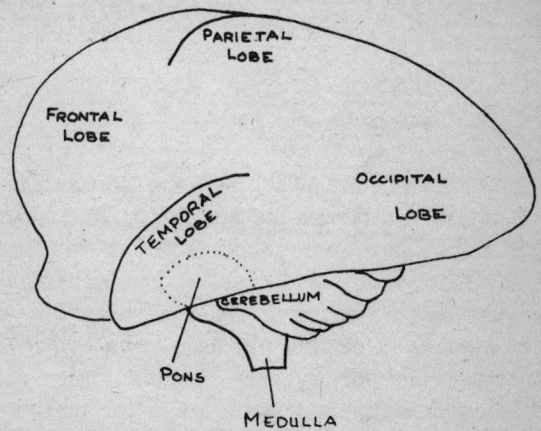

THE BRAIN—The Pons and the Medulla make up what is collectively called the Brain Stem. It is here that the mechanism controlling the processes of sleep are housed.

13

Drugs and Drug-Dependency Insomnia

If you've been taking pills to help you sleep you have probably been making a big mistake. A large number of insomniacs have caused themselves to have medical problems by taking sleeping pills. When an insomniac indicates that he has been taking sleeping pills, the sleep-specializing medical physician assumes that this patient has drug-dependency insomnia. Drug-dependency insomnia, the most frequently occurring type of insomnia, is an illness caused by a treatment. This illness is little known or understood by the medical profession.

A typical case of drug-dependency insomnia usually starts during a crisis. Let us look at the case of Ms. Branch. After many years of working herself through college and law school, the time has come for her to take the bar examination. Her success for the rest of her lifetime is probably dependent upon her passing this particular test. She was understandably worried,

Drugs and Drug-Dependency Insomnia

concerned, and began having difficulty sleeping at night prior to the examination. Because she was not sleeping well she found it difficult to study during the daytime hours. She consulted her doctor. Her doctor prescribed a reasonable dosage of a sleeping pill—a barbiturate—to be taken at bedtime every evening. Ms. Branch started taking the medication and found that it helped her disturbed sleep profoundly. As the examination time grew closer—approximately one week after she had begun taking the sleeping medication—she once again began to have difficulty sleeping, so she decided to take a double dose of the barbiturate. Full nights of sleep again returned. However, the cycle seemed to repeat itself, and again, one week later, the medication appeared not to be helping her any longer. She began to take three pills a night. Finally, she took her bar examination and the pressure lifted. The night of the examination she had a great deal of difficulty sleeping but decided that this was understandable since she was quite tense and apprehensive of the results. She continued to take her medication for a period of time until she received the results of her bar examination. She was most relieved to find that she had passed. That night she went to bed without swallowing her three sleeping pills. She could not sleep. In the middle of the night she got up and took three sleeping pills. After that she slept. Her difficulties with sleep continued, and she began to have terrible nightmares. She found it necessary to return to her sleeping-pill habit and began taking three pills once again nightly. She was not convinced that she had a terrible case of insomnia, and she was correct.

Ms. Branch came to me after two years of barbiturate swallowing. She was not sleeping well in spite of her high medication dosages nightly. Her sleep patterns were truly disturbed and abnormal. Throughout the previous two years she had taken as many as ten different types of sleeping pills, trying to find some variety that would help her to once again receive a good night's rest.

Ms. Branch's case is not unusual. Almost every hypnotic compound such as the barbiturate she was taking will cause, in time, the sort of condition that Ms. Branch developed. The listing at the end of this chapter indicates which common sleeping medications are hypnotic. Although hypnotics seem to be the worst type of sleeping draught to take, other drug preparations will also cause drug-dependency insomnia in time.

There is only one known treatment for drug-dependency insomnia—the patient must completely refrain from taking the drug. A physician's care is necessary and important during the drug withdrawal program. As the patient withdraws from the medication there is an excellent chance that he or she will develop horrible nightmares. It is not smart to try to stop taking the medication all at once. Rapid withdrawal will lead to even more severe and frightening nightmares and possible convulsive seizures. Patients who manage to withdraw from the drug's grasp do eventually sleep well again. Anyone who continues to take the barbiturates for years will not experience a good night's rest. Of all the patients I have treated for this disorder, I can honestly say that one-hundred percent of those who withdrew from drugs slept better and felt better after complete withdrawal. There are not many medical treatments which can boast such an excellent success score.

Drug-dependency insomnia can also be caused by

alcohol taken as a sleeping medication. The treatment is the same; complete withdrawal is necessary, although during this procedure violent nightmares might occur.

It is obvious that physicians prescribing these drugs are either unaware or uncaring of the consequences of taking them over a long period of time. As sleep research becomes one of the more popular fields of scientific inquiry, the problems connected with the ingestion of sleeping drugs will become better known to the general physician. But you now know about it. Stop taking those pills and find yourself a physician who understands that you have drug-dependency insomnia. You need treatment.

Statistics relating to drug-dependency insomnia are frightening. For every person hooked on hard narcotics there are approximately twelve barbiturate addicts in this country. The late Connecticut Senator Thomas Dodd stated in 1962, "A virtual epidemic of 'nice-drug' addiction is sweeping the country." Individuals in the United States pay about one million dollars a year for sedatives for which a prescription is required; they pay even more for over-the-counter sleeping medications, approximately $350 million a year. Over $250 million is spent on tranquilizers in the United States, and of course a great deal of alcohol is purchased and consumed to be used as a sleeping pill.

A serious problem with reliance upon these drugs is that one quickly develops a tolerance to the specific dosage being taken at any given time. The drug-taker suddenly realizes that the amount of medication she or he has been taking simply no longer works. So the dosage is increased. It is much as if you were drinking water in another country. When you first arrived in that country, the particular minerals in that area would affect your system and cause you to be ill, but after you drank the water for a month the mineral content would no longer bother your system and you would be as healthy as the natives who had lived there all their lives. The tolerance our bodies have of foreign and unknown ingestives is essentially a survival mechanism. Without it we would be ill a great deal more of the time than we are. A sleeping pill is essentially a toxin, and as a patient continues to ingest the toxin its effect slowly but surely begins to be less felt as the body adjusts to having what is essentially a poison within its system. Thus, the individual is forced to take more of the toxin or sleeping pill. This is a slow, gentle path that many people go down, and they are hooked on drugs before they even realize it.

Most individuals in the United States who are taking sleeping medications are not doing so because they are seeking thrills or because they wish to commit suicide. The usual reason for their taking this medication originally was that they wanted to sleep. A situation or schedule such as Ms. Branch's which causes tension is often the starting point for a barbiturate habit.

Are you taking a dangerous drug to help you sleep at present? You must remember that almost everyone at one time or another in their lives has difficulty sleeping. It is not necessary to "take something" to ensure you a good night's rest. If you don't sleep well for one or two nights, that is perfectly acceptable. These drugs are too dangerous to play around with.

Prior to the advent of barbiturates, physicians prescribed alcohol or "knock-out drops" to people having difficulty sleeping. Not everyone wanted to drink alcohol to help them sleep, while on the other hand, some enjoyed it a bit too much. Knock-out drugs—

usually chlorylhydrate or paraldehyde—tasted terrible and smelled even worse. So when barbiturates became available on the market they were immediately successful. Doctors started to prescribe pentobarbital, which is sold under the name Nembutal, and secobarbital, sold as Seconal. These two hypnotics are considered to be quick-acting and are effective for a short period of time against sleeplessness. There is no question that these two drugs can become addictive.

As physicians learned of the increasing nonmedical, addictive use of these barbiturates, they turned instead to newer types of drugs for insomnia, such as ethchlorbynol (Placidyl) and flurazepam (Dalmane). Nembutal and Seconal affected the central nervous system, and the new depressants do also. Unfortunately, the possibility of addiction is just as strong with the new drugs as it is with Nembutal and Seconal. The American Medical Association publishes a book called *AMA Drug Evaluations* which discusses these hypnotics and warns, "Long-term use of larger-than-usual therapeutic doses may result in psychic and physical dependence."

Certain drugs usually taken to ease anxiety and tension are also prescribed at times for insomnia. This group of prescription medications, considered to be "minor tranquilizers," includes Equanil, Miltown, Librium, and Valium, as well as many others. They are addictive.

But what about the sleeping medications one can buy over the counter, without a prescription? These sleep-aids and sedatives are not tranquilizers. Nor are they barbiturates. Sure-Sleep, Sleep-Eze, Dormin, Nite-Rest, and Nytol contain mainly antihistamines. Antihistamines really have nothing to do with helping an individual sleep; they are intended to prevent allergic reactions. The fact that they make some individuals drowsy when taken as an anti-allergenic, prompted manufacturers to promote them as a sleeping aid. Sure-Sleep also contains a bit of aspirin, as does Nytol. Some of these drugs—Nite-Rest, Sleep-Eze, and Sure-Sleep—contain scopolamine, or a form of scopolamine called hyoscine. Scopolamine is a mild sedative that comes from the plant belladonna. Actually the amount of scopolamine found in these over-the-counter sleep preparations is too insignificant to put anyone to sleep, except psychologically. There is no particular reason why scopolamine is used in conjunction with an antihistamine; the two together do not particularly induce sleep.

Also sold over the counter as sleeping aids is a group of medications which suggest that they will help the insomniac by relieving tension. The drug Compoz, which is advertized as "the largest-selling nonprescription sedative for temporary relief of simple nervous tension," will not, in fact, relieve anxiety and won't help anyone sleep either. Compoz contains not one but two antihistamines and scopolamine. Studies have proven that Compoz, with its antihistamines and scopolamine, is no more effective for reducing tension and aiding in sleep than the ingestion of aspirin would be.

The prescription medication chlordiazepoxide (Librium) does appear to help sleep problems. But it too is addictive and can cause drug-dependency insomnia. There *are* specific instances when an individual should take a medication for an insomnia-related problem. One must be sure, however, that the physician understands that these sleeping drugs can often cause more problems than they cure. Discuss this problem with your physician prior to beginning a sleeping-preparation regime, even with an over-the-counter drug, for the side-effects can be devastating.

Compoz is a fine example of a drug that causes uncomfortable side-effects. Blurred vision can result, and increased pressure in the eyes. The mouth may become dry and the patient may find it difficult to urinate. Individuals with glaucoma—and there are number of people walking around with this disease who do not know they have it—can be severely affected by the ingestion of Compoz.

Scopolamine, a common ingredient of sleeping medicines, can at times cause behavioral abnormalties. Although this reaction will usually only occur after prolonged use, obviously this is not a drug you should be taking to help you sleep. The amount of scopolamine contained in Compoz (0.15 milligrams) is actually smaller than the amount contained in a number of other medications. The drug with the highest amount of scopolamine is Sominex capsules (0.5 mg). Other medications containing high amounts of scopolamine are:

Nite-Rest	0.25 mg
San-Man	0.25 mg
Sominex tablets	0.25 mg
Sure-Sleep	0.2 mg
Seedate	0.125 mg
Sleep-Eze	0.125 mg

The drugs mentioned also contain antihistamines. As I have already indicated, there is absolutely no reason for an individual to take an antihistamine when he wishes to sleep, unless he happens to be suffering from hayfever at the same time. Aside from the fact that the antihistamines are not a sensible medication for insomnia, there are specific reasons why one should not take this type of medication unless absolutely necessary. The side-effects of antihistamines are a lack of coordination, blurred vision, a loss of appetite called anorexia, dizziness, rashes, changes in the composition of the blood, and sometimes frequent urination. These problems usually will not surface while the individual is taking only a small amount of antihistamines. However, they do crop up with larger-dose intake. Needless to say, a side-effect such as dizziness can be quite dangerous at a time, for example, when one is driving a car.

Antihistamines and scopolamine are promoted for insomnia and as hypnotics because they produce drowsiness when taken for treatment of allergic diseases. Also when one takes these drugs for the prevention of motion sickness, sleepiness sometimes results. But, to take a drug that is indicated for a specific illness so that its side-effects may help you sleep is foolhardy. Antihistamines affect the central nervous system, and might in fact help some individuals to sleep for a while. But a case of persistent chronic insomnia will not be touched by these drugs. If you still insist on taking these over-the-counter preparations, be sure that you follow the manufacturer's dosage recommendations. These drugs are probably safe if taken at the dosages specified on the package. But if you find that these amounts do not help you to sleep, do not take larger doses.

Drugs prescribed and taken for insomnia (including over-the-counter medications) are listed below. Of course, many of the drugs have similar ingredient-combinations. A number of them contain phenobarbital; about thirty include amphetamine sulfate. This list cannot be complete; new drugs are placed on the market constantly.

BARBITURATES

Alurate
Amytal
Butisol
Cabrital
Eskabarb
Evipal
Luminal
Mebaral
Medomin
Nembutal
Seconal
Sombulex
Stental
Tuinal
Veronal

NONBARBITURATE HYPNOTICS

Beta-Chlor
Bromural
Dalmane
Doriden
Dormal
En-Chlor
Felusels
Loryl
Noctec
Noludar
Paral
Placidyl
Quaalude
Taborea
Tindal
Valmid

NONPRESCRIPTIVE DRUGS

Alva-Tranquil
Compoz
Devarex
Dormin
Mr. Sleep
Neo-Nyte
Nervine
Nytol
San-Man
Sleep-Eze
Sominex
Somnicaps
Sure-Sleep

ANTIHISTAMINES AND HISTAMINE INHIBITORS

Benadryl
Eutonyl
Marplan
Monofen
Nardil

Parnate
Phenergan
Stinerval
Tanabe
Vistaril

ANTIDEPRESSANT DRUGS

Allegran
Aventyl
Elavil
Laroxyl
Norpramin

Pertofrane
Saroten
Tofranil
Tryptanol

MAJOR TRANQUILIZERS (antipsychotic drugs)

Aminazin
Ampliactil
Anatensol
Chlorpiprazin
Compazine
Decentan
Diopal
Eskazinyl
Fentazine
Jatroneural
Largactil
Malloryl
Mellaril
Melleretten
Nipodal
Penthoxate

Permitil
Phenergan
Prolixin
Protactil
Prozine
Serpasil
Sparine
Stelazine
Stemetil
Talofen
Temetil
Terfluzin
Thorazine
Tindal
Trancin
Triafon

MINOR TRANQUILIZERS (anti-anxiety drugs)

Atarax
Capla
Equanil
Librium

Meprospan
Miltown
Serax
Solacen

STIMULANTS (taken to stay awake)

Benzedrine
Desoxyephedrine
Desoxyn
Desyphed
Dexamyl
Dexedrine

Efroxine
Methedrine
No-Doz
Norodin
Sta-Wake
Syndrox

14

The Sleep Method—One Step to Sleep

We have now discussed the various types of insomnia and the reasons for them. Perhaps you have found that your anxiety over your inability to get what you consider to be a good night's sleep was inappropriate. As you studied the Sleep Questionnaire you filled out at the beginning of this book, we hope you gained insight into your particular problem and were perhaps able to solve it. Being overly concerned about the amount of sleep that you get will certainly not aid the problem. Perhaps you are one of those people who now realizes that the hours spent awake in the middle of the night can be put to useful purposes. We all have insomnia at one time or another in our lives. If you have problems bothering you, do not blame your unhappiness and inability to deal with the day ahead of you on insomnia. Perhaps the insomnia is the result of these other lingering problems and difficulties. Try to understand your own particular problem; it may well be that you are sleeping better already.

If your particular insomnia-related problem is so severe, intense, and chronic that it is essentially an illness, you should probably seek psychiatric and medical help. If your sleep patterns have changed drastically and are affecting your daily efficiency to the point where you are unable to function, seek medical assistance. Remember, however, that if you do consult a physician, do not assume that the doctor is aware of the dangers of drug therapy—primarily the possibility of addiction and drug-dependency insomnia. Be sure that the physician you visit is well aware of these particular problems and well-versed on insomnia-related illnesses. In other words, try to go to an expert on sleep problems.

There is no question that *an orderly routine* will help you sleep at night. Get in the habit of doing the same things every night prior to climbing into bed and you will find that your night's rest is more satisfying. Baths and showers are relaxing; if you have a sleep problem it makes sense to bathe prior to going to bed every night.

Do not catnap during the day. Remember that the time spent catnapping during the daylight hours must be added to the nighttime sleep period to present a full picture of your sleep patterns. If you want to sleep more soundly at night, it makes sense not to sleep during the day. No matter how tired you feel in the daylight hours, do not sleep.

Exercise regularly and moderately every night prior to going to bed. It might help you sleep better, and it certainly will benefit your overall physical condition.

Then there is the subject of *diet*.... We have come to the point in this book where I will explain to you my Sleep Method. It does not involve medication, and only involves exercise to the point I have indicated above; a bit of mild exercise prior to climbing into the bed does usually help an individual to sleep better. The Sleep Method involves rather what might be called a "natural sleeping pill." This type of sleep-inducer will not cause morning-after hangover and drowsiness and helps to induce a healthy, normal slumber.

We all know how sleepy we get after a large holiday dinner, such as at Thanksgiving time. There is a medical, scientifically proven reason for this—*tryptophan* (pronounced TRIP-tow-fan). Tryptophan is an amino acid—a protein—and is found in many foods.

In the past it was assumed that people became sleepy after ingesting a large amount of food because the blood would leave the brain and go to the gut after heavy eating, and the lack of the usual amount of blood within the head would cause drowsiness. However, this has never been proven as being correct. In fact, most research physicians thought the theory was rather unsound. Actually, something specific does happen within the brain after eating a heavy meal. As an individual eats foods containing tryptophan, the protein is changed into another substance containing *serotonin*. Serotonin is a biochemical that is known to be present in the brain, and scientists have known for quite some time that it has a connection with regulating sleep patterns. In some way not clearly understood by researchers, serotonin, which is the result of eating the protein tryptophan, triggers sleep naturally. Needless to say, this is a much superior method for inducing sleep than barbiturates. The fact is, tryptophan appears to produce a much more normal restful sleep than any known sleeping medications manage to do.

A number of studies have been completed involving tryptophan, and the evidence is that the subjects slept more soundly and peacefully after ingesting tryptophan than they did after any other known sleep-inducer. This determination was made from all-night brain-wave recordings as well as from interviews with the subjects when they awoke.

The most interesting thing about tryptophan is that it is found in meats, milks, and cheese and is quite plentiful. Researchers at Boston's Tufts-New England Medical Center and at Stanford University in California, have found that it takes only a small amount of tryptophan to cut the usually required amount of time lying in bed prior to falling asleep in half.

Tryptophan appears to act as a natural sedative when taken in the proper dose. Studies done by Dr. Clinton Brown, of Johns Hopkins University, and Dr. Althea Wagman, of the Maryland Psychiatric Research Center, indicate that individuals who spent about one hour falling to sleep and had been having insomnious-type problems for a number of years, cut this time to only one-half hour after eating foods containing tryptophan. This change took place within a period of two weeks. The twelve female subjects studied in this particular test had their sleep patterns monitored electronically during this period of time. The tracings showed that they slept more soundly after ingesting tryptophan. In addition, these females slept an average of forty-five minutes longer than they did prior to the tryptophan ingestion.

No one really understands how tryptophan works. The production of serotonin and the effect of serotonin upon the sleep center within the brain is not completely understood. But one thing is—tryptophan helps insomniacs. And of course one of the greatest advantages of tryptophan is that it is not addicting, it cannot cause coma or death taken in large doses, and your body naturally needs and uses the protein. You will not be introducing a toxic substance into your system.

All of the studies done with tryptophan also included the introduction of a placebo in a control group as well. In other words, the scientists setting up the tests grouped the individuals being tested into two specific groups, which were as alike as humanly possible. Each group had the same number of males and females, both groups had people of identical ages, health, background, and occupation. One of these two groups received the tryptophan night after night and their brainwaves were studied. The other group received a placebo, or a phoney tryptophan, usually made of sugar, and neither group knew which was receiving the drug being tested and which was receiving the placebo. In fact, even the researchers did not know which group was which until all of the data and information was collected and compiled and the results were charted. One group was obviously more successful at getting to sleep and staying asleep than the other. The researchers did not look to see which group had taken the placebo and which had ingested tryptophan until it was determined which group was more successful at sleep. When the results were in, it was clear that tryptophan was helping people to sleep.

One of the nicest things about tryptophan is that you do not have to go to your doctor for a prescription, and you do not have to go to your drugstore to buy it. It occurs naturally in a number of foods which you normally eat. In the past, sleep physicians thought that milk at bedtime seemed to help certain people sleep because of a psychological association with their mothers and their babyhood, rather than any scientifically credible reason. They are now having to admit that they were wrong. Milk happens to contain a goodly amount of tryptophan.

Researchers have differing opinions as to how much tryptophan it is necessary to take prior to going to bed. I recommend to my patients that they ingest about *one gram of tryptophan at least one-half hour, but not more than one hour, prior to going to bed.* The following chart lists the amount of tryptophan found in a variety of foods and indicates the number of grams—a weight measure—within each individual foodstuff. To give you a basis of comparison, let me point out that one raisin weighs one gram.

$$1 \text{ gram} = 1/28\text{th ounce}$$
$$1 \text{ raisin} = 1 \text{ gram}$$
$$28 \text{ raisins} = 1 \text{ ounce}$$

While there is no question that tryptophan is a natural sleep inducer that will help you to fall asleep and sleep well during the night, perhaps the true deliverance from your insomnia lies within yourself. You must adhere to a regular schedule, you should exercise daily, preferably in the evening, and you should do the same specific relaxing activities every evening prior to bedtime. My method is most effective, however, if ultimate control of your insomnia is within your will. Although as you get older you will sleep less heavily and perhaps meet with some minor sleep problems, and through all during your life tense situations, unhappiness, and anxiety will affect your sleep patterns, the fact of the matter is, you are the one who really controls how you sleep. You must teach yourself to relax,

Number of Grams of Tryptophan per 4-Ounce Serving

Non-fat dried milk	.5 grams
Peanut butter	.4
Peanuts	.4
Eggs	.2
Leg of lamb	.2
Chicken	.3
Fish	.2
Liver	.3
White bread	.1
Shredded wheat	.1
Oatmeal	.2
Puffed rice	.5
Puffed oats, corn, or rye	.2
Bananas	.2
Grapefruit	.01
Oranges, or orange juice	.03
Lima beans	.5
String beans	.2
Cauliflower	.3
Spinach	.4
Summer squash	.05
Celery	.1
Corn	.1
Onions	.2

to ignore sounds while you are sleeping, and you must stop worrying about your lack of sleep. Your whole being must experience a sense of well-being, and this feeling of satisfaction must be present not only during your waking hours but also while you are asleep.

15

The Alpha-State—Mastering Your Mind

You are in charge of your mind; there is no question about that. And since this is true it stands to reason that your problems with insomnia are to a large part solvable by yourself alone, without any outside influences. You have the power to control how well or how poorly you sleep. You must learn to use that ability and profit from it. The payoff will be pleasant evenings of rest.

We have all heard of the feats performed by yogis in India. Individuals have been studied who could make themselves perspire on their foreheads whenever they decided to. These people have learned to raise the temperature of their skins and elevate their heartbeats whenever they desire. There are individuals who can control their heartbeats and can, in fact, stop their hearts from beating. Certain specific muscles are contracted, resulting in a decreased flow of blood to the heart and the pulse becomes impossible to feel. At the same time the blood-pressure lowers. The philosophy of yoga includes breathing exercises which can bring you to the point where your respiration can be completely controlled by you. During a yogi's cross-legged meditation, he experiences complete and deliberate relaxation throughout his whole system. Yogis can remain still for hours while in this relaxed state. They appear to hear nothing and can not be distracted as they meditate. Their muscular relaxation is almost identical to that of a sleeper during a REM sleep dream period. In fact, the yogi discipline—involving relaxed breathing, muscles, posture, and thinking—results in the attainment of a state that performs the functions a person would usually have to sleep to get the advantage of.

The Zen Buddhists—also meditators—sit for long hours in the lotus position, with their eyes looking down at a specific spot on the ground. They claim to attain a sense of enlightenment during this type of closely disciplined meditation. Breathing is controlled by themselves so that it is regular and rhythmic, and these people have been known to sit in a lotus position and meditate for many hours or days without sleep, although they are experiencing a form of sleep by holding themselves right at the point prior to sleep, when the whole system relaxes. This condition also occurs as a person begins to awaken, and it is difficult to differentiate between sleeping and waking at this point during an individual's physiological condition.

There are people who are able to place themselves in what we now call the alpha-state—just as the Zen Buddhists and yogis are able to do—at will. In addition, these individuals are able to completely control

The Alpha-State—Mastering Your Mind

when they are in the alpha-state and when they wish to emerge from it. It is probably true that all of us enter the alpha-state several times during each day, but we are unaware of it. Most people do not have any clear idea regarding the alpha-state and what it is exactly. It is a difficult sensation to describe and identify.

The usual method of identifying when an individual is in the alpha-state is via instrumentation hooked up to the person's head. When the person reaches the alpha-state a certain sound is emitted from the machine. Yet I have found it is possible to enter the alpha-state without purchasing any specific devices. It is a good idea for you to learn to enter this state, because it is an unusually relaxed attitude to enter. Being able to induce the alpha-state will help you to relax and sleep better. Sit back in a comfortable chair, in a quiet room, with no distractions, and put your feet up on a footstool. Relax completely. Let your mind think about all your muscles relaxing.... Close your eyes and roll your eyes back up into your head several times. As you do this you should feel a muscular loosening around your forehead and temples. To physically relax the rest of the muscles of your scalp and ears, roll your eyes up into your head once again. During this procedure you should be feeling a pleasurable, vacant sort of serenity. You will be right on the edge between being awake and being asleep. In a recently publicized case, an American woman placed herself in alpha-state—or as she put it, meditated—for five days. She did not sleep during this period of time and yet the psychiatrist who monitored this process stated that she seemed refreshed and relaxed at the end of the five-day period.

The alpha-state has been touted as a difficult-to-learn procedure. However, if you have just followed my directions carefully and felt yourself to be extremely relaxed, you may well have been experiencing the alpha-state. The more you practice this alpha-relaxation, the better your chances are of being able to control it and experience it whenever you desire. You will find that if you are busy and tense during the day, you can lean back in your chair and experience the alpha-state even for as little as thirty seconds and feel relaxed when you open your eyes once again.

It is even possible to get a "feeling" for the alpha-state by rolling your eyes back into your head while you are awake. Try it. You can immediately feel the loosening of muscles around the eyes. When you close your eyes, completely relax all of your 639 muscles, and experience the alpha-state, you are very close to being in the same situation as you are in the nighttime when you dream during REM sleep. Although it has not been definitely proven, I firmly believe—due to my own personal experiences—that the alpha-state is as much a muscle manipulation as it is a frame of mind. This statement will undoubtedly upset individuals who feel that there is a great depth of meaning within the alpha experience. I, however, consider it to be wonderful news. People who can place themselves in the alpha-state find that they are more relaxed and less tense than they were prior to discovering this ability. There is no question in my mind that insomniacs will be helped by practicing the alpha-state during the day and at bedtime.

Incidentally, another great help for insomniacs is to read a book about insomnia at bedtime! There is nothing that is more sleep-inducing, in my opinion, than letting your mind play with the various stages of sleep, descriptions of sleep periods, and general discussions concerning sleep. If all else fails, pick this book up and start reading it. I guarantee you'll be asleep shortly thereafter.

16

The Cloud of Sleep

At night we feel a wave of change overcome us. Our eyes become functionally blind and our brains cease to deliver sights, sounds, and smells. We tend to fall away from the present world and we drift, feeling subtle moods ... we are barely within the fragile area defining the difference between awakeness and sleep. The soft progression into sleep can be changed suddenly if, as we lie in the darkness, we suppose for instance that we hear someone opening a window in the downstairs living-room. Suddenly, from the depths of our thinking minds there is a communication immediately sent to the brain and then throughout our being. Our heartbeats increase and our blood fills with adrenaline. Our muscles are ready to move. But then we seem to begin to fall once again into the cloudlike softness and soothing darkness and warmth, and the caution and alarm we felt a moment before subsides.

Though we are like a feather falling through the air as we sink down through sleep, our brain cells do not

The Cloud of Sleep

stop their work. They are constantly alert and are on guard for ominous threats. Anything new might cause our brain cells to sharpen and become excited, although if whatever arouses them continues repetitiously they will become accustomed to it quite quickly. For example, a household heating system or air-conditioner, although continuously transmitting noises, will be ignored by the brain cells. In fact, we may become awakened if the sound ceases.

And so our nocturnal journey continues ... we float down and rise up ... down and up, .. down toward consciousness and then down again to a new level. Our flotations are never exactly the same at any level on any given night. Our brains act differently throughout each shift in each ascent and descent. We sleep. We may be unhappy, or our voices may ring out with laughter. If we are asked a question, we may answer. Our minds might wander and we might babble. Perhaps we will stand up, get out of bed, and walk around the room; our sleeping expressions might contain fear or happiness. This is sleep. Why?

Primitive people believed naively that the very soul was freed in sleep and wandered and talked with the spiritual environment of the nighttime. As scientists started to study sleep, they looked to the body for understanding. As long ago as the sixth century B.C. the Greeks thought that sleep was the result of blood rushing to the body and leaving the mind in an anemic and undernourished state. Although this has been proven to be untrue, there are unusual differences in our circulatory systems and within our brain as we sleep. The arteries within our necks experience pressure changes and this seems to have an influence on the brain and its state of sleep or wakefulness.

Another theory was that the brain was starved of

oxygen during sleep, but this has been proven to be untrue. In actuality, the brain holds a high level of oxygenation during sleep. The activities of the muscles and other bodily functions were thought to cause the body to become fatigued to the point where the tiredness would become overpowering. The brain would then tell the body to become refreshed. Many different organs of the body have been thought to be influential in the phenomenon of sleep and today we believe that a large number of our organs do indeed have an effect upon the beginning and continuation of sleep patterns. This is probably because of the effect of the organs upon our brain cells.

More recently—within the past thirty years—researchers seem to have decided to study the brain itself, rather than the whole being, in connection with sleep research. There are two specific networks of nerve cells paralleling the spinal cord and entering various areas of the brain. If these brain cells are shocked or excited by chemicals, evidently one of the two networks of nerve cells will cause sleep and the other will induce waking.

One of the biggest problems connected with the study and understanding of sleep has been that the scientists looking into the aspects of sleep were usually, necessarily, trained in only one discipline and lacked knowledge of the work connected with sleeping being done by scientists in other disciplines. As each scientist had a different focus of attention—one might be interested in dreams, while another might be interested in the cardiovascular system—it was really quite difficult for any single scientist to have at his or her disposal enough information and data to gain a clear understanding of the phenomenon of sleep.

The Cloud of Sleep

Things have changed within the past ten years, however. Sleep scientists have started communicating with one another and sharing their information. It is now possible for the researchers who are studying, for example, the cardiovascular system to understand the theory of dream content, stomach changes, and drug-induced insomnia as well. Although science has made great strides recently in the area of sleep, the fact of the matter is, we still don't know what sleep is.

Yet the average citizen in the United States knows that when she or he falls asleep there is not merely a loss of consciousness—some other things are going on as well. The individual can feel the transition from one level of sleep to another and does experience fleeting, short dreams and thoughts. A muscle spasm is noticed; a muscular-relaxation feeling then envelops the person. The breathing changes and the individual can recognize this. The third and fourth stages of sleep slowly overcome the person.

It is not possible to stay within the third and fourth stages of sleep for long. A rise toward the surface of wakefulness will take approximately one and a half hours. During this period (what we call REM sleep) about ten minutes of stormy dreaming might occur. One individual might begin to grind teeth; a male might experience an erection. Eye movements will be noticeable and breathing will be somewhat less than smooth. The beginning dream of the night will often contain remnants of the past day's activities and will slowly disappear as the person goes into the depths of quiet sleep.

This trance-like stage might cause the individual to speak or sit up and at times get out of bed. After this first REM sleep of the night, about an hour and a half will go by. The sleeper will then begin to breathe on an irregular basis once again, and the pulse will race. This next dream episode will probably contain sensations and experiences not related to the previous day. There is a good chance that, in fact, these dreams will not be concerned with the daily experiences at all.

Another six hours of sleep will transpire. The dream stage will then again take place, and at this time the dreamer will have extremely vivid, colorful, sensual, and sexual dreams. Circumstance and reason will now have no place in these dreams. There is a good chance that the individual will experience another intense dream period prior to awakening. The only possible dream that will be remembered in the morning will be the last one.

Although the dreamer will have been for a number of hours in a dark, misty, unfathomable state, she or he knows that this experience is not—as was believed in earlier times—a form of death. Yet we do not know really why this quiet period overtakes us. It happens every day to every human being and every animal, but we simply do not know why. Evolutionists believe that the first cellular life on our planet had close ties and relationships with the sun and required solar energy to survive. Without daylight these single-celled organisms would die. These one-celled animals evolved into creatures of the sea and, it is believed by many, incorporated the tides (affected by the moon's gravity) and the rhythms of the oceans into their existence. Perhaps our periods of sleep and awakening may in some way be a remnant of what these single-celled beings required for life. Perhaps a clock within our minds dictates our sleep periods and the time we are awake. There are many different cycles within the human organisms that follow a daily pattern. Perhaps rather than the timer being within our brains, we *are* in essence the clock itself. Maybe our very flesh has a rhythm to it. The organs of our bodies and the workings of our systems do seem to fluctuate in a certain specific way on a twenty-four-hour basis. When we are ill our symptoms show a cyclical pattern as well. When we travel in a jet our bodies are upset because of the change in time zone. We are made uncomfortable, tired, and "hung-over." If we continue in this pattern for a long period of time we begin to suffer the same sorts of problems as night-workers, stewardesses, and pilots are familiar with. This problem is not eliminated for people who reverse their daytime and nighttime activities. Although it would seem that these individuals would be able to become essentially nocturnal beings, they often suffer from psychological upsets as well as disturbed sleep patterns.

There is no longer any question that there are certain timing devices within us that we must acknowledge and credit with importance. When we try to go against our bodily rhythms we suffer for it. On the other hand, if we work with our own particular bodily fluctuations we can learn to reach new heights of physical and mental capabilities. It appears that there are times when certain sorts of activities will be more effectual, both mental and physical. Perhaps there are certain periods when it would be more sensible to receive medical attention than at others. There is a possibility that the treatment might be more effective if it fits in with one's personal clocking device.

We would all like to know how the darkness and the daylight, love, laughter, and sorrow, and various foods affect our bodies' rhythms. There has been no other time throughout history that it was so possible to expect to find the answers to these rather ultimate questions. Perhaps these answers will be looked upon with disfavor by certain individuals because they will surely indicate that the human being has certain specific limitations in body and mind. There are many people who wish to be able to sleep when they choose, and for the amount of time that they desire; I myself would be happier if I only had to sleep say two nights a week rather than seven. Would you be pleased to be able to take a pill once a day rather than to sleep at night? Perhaps not. There are many individuals, however, who do wish that they could manipulate their sleep patterns for their own convenience.

At a time when many people wish that they could completely eliminate sleep from the necessities of life, scientists are proving more and more clearly that one absolutely cannot do without slumber. There are inherent dangers in a lack of sleep, and we must all accept the fact that nightly regular sleep is important to our general well-being. When we do not accept this fact and fight it, we find that our bodies and minds begin to deteriorate quite rapidly. One begins to become an unreliable individual, although at times one can appear to be quite clever, alert and sharp. There is the tendency towards erratic behavior during times of sleep deprivation. In fact, the individual who is in need of sleep will often essentially sleep on his feet for short periods of time. If one has an alcoholic beverage when in need of sleep, the reaction to the alcohol will be much more severe than if it were consumed when the individual was well-rested. Hallucinations might occur and the person might become psychotic for short periods of time. Various unusual sensations will overtake the body in waves. Certain types of individuals such as the mentally ill, epileptics, and sufferers of narcolepsy often are insomniacs, and they seem to suffer more than the average individual does when they are lacking in restful slumber.

There are very few people who actually try not to sleep by skipping one night of sleep out of every two. But there are in fact many individuals who try to cut down by an hour or so the amount of daily sleep their bodies seem to require. These people will suffer for this in the end. The quality of the rest experienced during the shortened night is different than if one were to sleep the number of hours that his or her body needs. Sleep loss affects the mind. There is no drug substitute for it and we probably will never find one.

17

The Electric Dormitory

New things are happening in the treatment of insomnia; ideas which were futuristic only a few years ago are now being used to help insomniacs. Unfortunately, the number of insomniacs that can receive help in clinics, hospitals, and research institutions is minute in comparison to the number of people suffering from this particular problem. There are ways to treat, diagnose, and probably cure the severe insomniac —and I am speaking here of individuals who have a medical problem—but unfortunately the facilities that must be available to help these individuals are expensive and there are very few of them available in this country at present.

Yet people spend and spend and spend for drugs related to insomnia: tranquilizers, sedatives, and hypnotics. The cost of insomnia is much greater than this, however. One must take into account the number of accidents on the roads caused by people who lack proper rest, and we must also consider the faulty decisions made by businessmen, irritability towards children by parents, and drug-dependency.

It is possible in this country to walk into a drug store and purchase many different remedies for insomnia. Doctors are as much at fault regarding the present situation as is anyone. Physicians will often prescribe a medication for treatment with barely any thought as to the consequences, yet if the patient were suffering from a stomach disorder they would never presume to prescribe in such a haphazard manner. The result is that new problems and illnesses are created rather than the original malady cured.

An institution that would help solve these problems and disseminate sleep knowledge to general physicians as well would be a sleep clinic. Many researchers delving into the phenomenon of sleep feel that every major hospital in the country should have a sleep clinic available to its patients. This clinic would be essentially a diagnostic place; people with sleep problems could go there and find out exactly what was causing them. These sleep clinics could be set up in such a way that parents could stay with their children and perhaps husbands with their wives. The period of study usually required for a sleep problem is at least two or three nights and sometimes longer; during this period of time the patient would be checked by a medical staff member and a psychiatric worker. The diet of the patient could be controlled; for example, no coffee, tea, or other stimulants would be allowed during the daytime. In addition, the protein tryptophan would be given in large doses throughout the day. The individual would be wired up prior to going to sleep and would be studied electronically throughout the night.

People often think that they are not sleeping when they are. The records that would be obtained in a sleep clinic such as this would tell the real story. This would be helpful to the doctors as well as to the patients themselves. A recent study at the University of Florida indicated that of the twenty-some patients who complained of sleeping practically not at all during the night, almost all of them were sleeping a reasonable number of hours. The problem here was that their sleep was abnormal, *i.e.*, it was fitful, there was a great deal of difficulty in falling sleep initially, and there were frequent periods of awakening throughout the night. Individuals with problems such as this give researchers a clearer picture of what "normal" and "abnormal" sleep really are. So every patient studied within the sleep laboratory would be adding research data for sleep scientists to study; the patient would in addition be finding out precisely what he or she was doing throughout the night.

Patients at a sleep clinic would also be helped via a sensible diagnosis of their problems—the physicians and researchers could decide on the appropriate therapy for the individual.

Other countries such as Israel and Austria have a number of small sleep clinics scattered throughout the countryside. In the United States there is a sleep clinic which was opened in 1969 in Los Angeles at the Cedars-Sinai Medical Center. One of the techniques used at these clinics is electrical stimulation, or electrosleep. Although a number of these institutions unfortunately fail to delve deeply enough into the diagnostic end of insomnia prior to treating the patient, their reports of success via electro-sleep are interesting and perhaps encouraging. The clinics in Israel, Austria, and a few of those in England, Germany, and Russia, as well as the Los Angeles establishment, are treating their patients with a form of shock treatment, essentially an electric tranquilizer, which transmits a shock to the brain. While it does not necessarily induce sleep at that point, it seems to have the effect—according to reports—of "loosening up" the insomniac and relaxing him to the point where he will be able to experience more normal sleep patterns. The reports indicate that patients feel alert and awake after this therapy in contrast with individuals who go through shock therapy for psychiatric problems. One researcher described them as looking as if they had just awakened from a long night's restful sleep.

This shock treatment is accomplished with electrodes attached behind the ears and on the head which transmit impulses to the brain. The patient does not feel this, or if he does experience something, it is simply a slight tingling sensation. Although these pulses transmitted to the brain of the patient are quite weak, they do affect the brain cells and they establish a specific rhythm. Their effect upon the brain is somewhat close to the effect of an anesthesia. This technique is called the Electroson technique. Researchers who have experimented with it in the United States have found that there are noted changes in blood pressure, heart beat, and breathing, and the patients indicated that they did feel calmer and more relaxed as a result of the treatment. Only about half of the people within this experiment actually fell asleep, but practically all of them did seem to have some sort of a post-experiment tranquility.

People suffering from muscle spasms have also been treated with the Electroson method, and it seemed to help them. However, I must point out that much of the literature on this method was derived from Russian scientists and their data and compilation are skimpy although their enthusiasm is prolific. Research revolving around the Electroson technique is presently continuing in the United States, and within the next few years we should have a clearer picture of its effects as well as its defects.

As often happens with a new treatment, a number of physicians felt that Electroson therapy could be utilized for patients suffering from a variety of ailments, from schizophrenia to eczema to toxemia to ulcers. Although it does seem to have some relaxant qualities and a number of these ailments do relate directly or indirectly to emotional make-up and stress, not enough data has yet been compiled to indicate whether Electroson does indeed significantly help these individuals. The Electroson method is also being tried on patients suffering from illnesses relating to the central nervous system.

The Electroson treatment delivers impulses to the brain; a new technique being tested at present receives messages from the brain instead. The technique utilizes a device that is essentially an alarm clock which is portable and is in collusion with one's brain waves. This clock would be connected to the head. The delightfulness of the alarm would be that it would never ring at a time when it was difficult for an individual to awaken! Brain waves would be delivered to the clock which would analyze them and decide when a person was on the threshold of awakening. This might help insomniacs who seem to wake up at what is an abnormal time and perhaps would induce them to arise at the point when their bodies were best suited to it. This portable alarm clock is now being engineered so that it will not have to be directly connected by wires to the person that it is monitoring. All this might sound rather far-fetched and futuristic, but I would guess that within the next ten years these portable alarm clocks will be available to the average American.

We are all used to consulting our watches for clues as to when we should do certain specific daily activities such as getting ready for bed. Imagine a clock that would be geared to our inner systems that would truly tell us the best time to recline for our daily rest.

As we discuss new techniques and methods for treating the insomniac, let me once again remind you that you must never toy irresponsibly with your sleep pattern. To interfere with normal sleep is dangerous. We tend to think of sleep as something which we will partake of when it is to our convenience and then we often complain of having difficulty sleeping. Much of the insomnia suffered by people in the United States is of their own doing—we often push ourselves for too long and too far until we are close to the point of exhaustion. Happy, healthy individuals make a place for their sleep time. To be rested during the daytime after a comfortable night's slumber enhances the chance of a general sense of well-being throughout the daylight hours.

Bibliography

Tremendous advances leading toward a deeper understanding of sleep and insomnia have been made in the past several decades.

I have carefully compiled an extensive bibliography of books and articles, written for sleep scientists and laypeople, concerning the phenomenon of sleep. Ask your librarian for help in obtaining the articles which have appeared in scholarly journals. Ph.D. theses (doctoral dissertations) may be obtained by written order to: Xerox Ph.D. Service, Northwestern University, Evanston, Illinois. Continue to read about sleep; it's a large hunk of your life and highly interesting.

Abstracts of the Association for the Psychophysiological Study of Sleep, *Psychophysiology* 4(3), 1967, 1968.

Adams, R. D., Sleep and its abnormalities. In *Principles of Internal Medicine*, vol. I, ed. T. R. Harrison. McGraw-Hill, 1958.

Agnew, H. W., and Webb, W. B., The sleep patterns of long and short sleepers. Reprint J. Hillis Miller Health Center, April 6, 1967.

Agnew, H. W., Jr., Webb, W. B., and Williams, R. L., Comparison of Stage IV and I—REM sleep deprivation. *Perceptual and Motor Skills* 24:851–858, 1967.

Amadeo, M., and Gomez, E., Eye movements and dreaming in subjects with lifelong blindness. *Association for the Psychophysiological Study of Sleep*, Palo Alto, 1964.

Antrobus, J. S., Dement, W. C., and Fisher, C., Patterns of dreaming and dream recall: EEG study. *Journal of Abnormal Social Psychology* 69:341, 1964.

Aschoff, J., Circadian rhythms in man. *Science* 148, June 11, 1965.

Aserinsky, E., Brainwave pattern during the rapid eye movement period of sleep. *The Physiologist* 8:104, 1965.

Aston, R., and Hibbeln, P., Induced hypersensitivity to barbital in the female rat. *Science* 157:1463–1464, September 22, 1967.

Baekeland, F., Lasky, R., and Koulack, D., Effects of a stressful presleep experience on electroencephalograph-recorded sleep. *Psychophysiology*, 1968.

Baldridge, B. J., Whitman, R. M., and Kramer, M., The concurrence of fine muscle activity and rapid eye movement sleep. *Psychosomatic Medicine* 27:19–26, 1965.

Barber, B., *Drugs and Society*. Troy, N.Y.: Russell Sage Foundation, 1968.

Barber, T., Sleep and hypnosis: a reappraisal. *Journal of Clinical Experimental Hypnosis* 4:141–59, 1956.

Berger, R. J., Experimental modification of dream content by meaningful visual stimuli. *British Journal of Psychiatry* 109:722–740, 1963.

Berger, R. J., and Oswald, I., Eye movements during active and passive dreams. *Science* 137:601, 1962.

Berger, R. J., Olley, P., and Oswald, I., The EEG, eye movements and dreams of the blind. *Quarterly Journal of Experimental Psychology* 14:183, 1962.

Berlucchi, G., Callosal activity during sleep and wakefulness. *Association for the Psychophysiological Study of Sleep*, Washington, D.C., 1965.

Berrill, N. J., Living clocks. *Atlantic Monthly*, December, 1963.

Biological Clocks, Cold Spring Harbor Symposia on Quantitative Biology, Vol. xxv, The Biological Laboratory, Cold Spring Harbor, L. I., New York, 1960.

Bokert, E., Effects of Thirst and a Meaningfully Related Auditory Stimulus on Dream Reports. Unpublished Ph.D. thesis, New York University, 1965.

Brierley, N., *Learn While You Sleep*, London: Ward Lock & Co., Ltd., 1965.

Brill, A. A. (ed.), *The Basic Writings of Sigmund Freud*. New York: Modern Library, 1938.

Broughton, R. J., Sleep disorders: disorders of arousal? *Science*, 159:3819, 1070–78, 1968.

Brower, B., America's sleeping sickness—staying awake. *The New York Times Magazine*, October 15, 1961.

Brown, B., Shryne, J., and Dell, M., Relationship between personality-behavior characteristics and the sleep-dream cycle in cats. *Association for the Psychophysiological Study of Sleep*, Palo Alto, 1964.

Caspers, H., On steady potential shifts during various stages of sleep. *Neurophysiologie des Etats des Sommeil*. Editions du Centre National de la Recherche Scientifique, Paris, 1965.

Clarke, A. C., Sleep no more. *Holiday*, December, 1958.

Cohen, H. D., Shapiro, A., and Goodenough, D. R., The EEG during stage 4 sleep talking. *Association for the Psychophysiological Study of Sleep*, Washington, D.C., 1965.

Current Research on Sleep and Dreams. U.S. Dept. of Health, Education, and Welfare, U.S. Public Health Service, National Institute of Mental Health, Bethesda, Md. 1965.

Davidson, B., The thrill pill menace. *The Saturday Evening Post*, December 4, 1965.

De La Mare, W., *Behold This Dreamer!* New York: Knopf, 1939.

Dement, W. C., Dream recall and eye movements during sleep in schizophrenics and normals. *Journal of Nervous Mental Disorders* 122:263, 1955.

———, The effect of dream deprivation. *Science* 131:1705, 1960.

———, Experimental dream studies. In *Science and Psychoanalysis* 7:129–184, ed. J. Masserman; Grune & Stratton, 1964.

———, Recent studies on the biological role of rapid eye movement sleep. *American Journal of Psychiatry.* 122:404, 1965.

Dement, W. C., and Wolpert, E. A., The relationship of eye movement, body motility, and external stimuli to dream content. *Journal of Experimental Psychology* 55:543–553, 1958.

Deutsch, A., *The Shame of the States.* New York: Harcourt, Brace & World, 1948.

Diamond, E., *The Science of Dreams.* New York: McFadden-Bartell, 1963.

———, Long day's journey into the insomniac's night. *The New York Times Magazine*, p. 31, October 1, 1967.

Douthwaite, A. H., Sleeplessness better than drug abuse.... *British Medical Journal*, July 17, 1954.

Dunlap, K., *Habits, Their Making and Unmaking.* New York: Liveright, 1932.

Erickson, C. K., Sleep aids and other O-T-C sedatives in Handbook of Non-Prescription Drugs. *Journal of the American Pharmaceutical Association*, ed. G. B. Griffenhagen, 1967.

Essig, C. F., Newer sedative drugs that cause states of intoxication and dependence of barbiturate type. *Journal of the American Medical Association*, 196:714–717, May 23, 1966.

Feinberg, I., Koresko, R. L., Heller, N., and Steinberg, H. R., Unusually high dream time in an hallucinating patient. *American Journal of Psychiatry* 121:10, April, 1965.

Fischgold, H., Lavernhe, J., and Blanc, J., Sleep, insomnia and sleep debt. *Medical Press*, February 18, 1967.

Fisher, C., Gross, J., and Zuch, J., A cycle of penile erections synchronous with dreaming (REM) sleep. *Archives of General Psychiatry*. 12:29, 1965.

Fisher, C., *Dreaming and Sexuality*. New York: International Universities Press, 1966.

Fisher, C., Byrne, J. V., and Edwards, A., NREM and REM nightmares. *Psychophysiology*, September, 1968.

Fiss, H., and Ellman, S. J., The effects of REM sleep interruption on the sleep cycle. *Association for the Psychophysiological Study of Sleep*, 1968.

Freud, S., *The Interpretation of Dreams*. Science Editions, New York: John Wiley & Sons, 1960.

Fromm, E., *The Forgotten Language*. New York: Holt, Rinehart & Winston, 1951.

Foulkes, D., Dream reports from different stages of sleep. *Journal of Abnormal Social Psychology* 65:14–25, 1962.

———, *The Psychology of Sleep*. Scribner's, New York, 1966.

———, Dreams of the male child: four case studies. *Journal of Child Psychology and Psychiatry*, 1968.

Foulkes, D., and Vogel, G., Mental activity at sleep onset. *Journal of Abnormal Psychology* 70:231–243, 1965.

Foulkes, D., Spear, P. S., and Symonds, J. D., Individual differences in mental activity at sleep onset. *Journal of Abnormal Psychology* 71:280–286, 1966.

Foulkes, D., Pivik, T., Ahrens, J. B., and Swanson, E. M., Effects of "dream deprivation" on dream content: an attempted cross-night replication. *Journal of Abnormal Psychology*, in press.

Galton, L., The best time to work. *The New York Times Magazine*, November 5, 1961.

Giles, L., *Sleep*. Indianapolis, Ind.: Bobbs-Merrill, 1938.

Goodenough, D. R., Cyclical fluctuations in sleep depth and eye-movement activity during the course of natural sleep. *Canadian Psychiatric Journal* 8:406–408, 1963.

Goodenough, D. R., Shapiro, A., Holden, M., and Steinschriber, L., A comparison of "dreamers" and "nondreamers": eye movements, electroencephalograms, and the recall of dreams. *Journal of Abnormal Social Psychology* 62:295–302, 1959.

Green, W. J., The effect of LSD on the sleep-dream cycle. *Journal of Nervous Mental Disorders* 140:417–426, 1965.

Greenberg, R., Dream interruption insomnia. *Journal of Nervous Mental Disorders* 144(1):18–21, 1967.

Greenberg, R., and Pearlman, C., *Delerium tremens* and dreaming. *American Journal of Psychiatry* 124:2, August, 1967.

———, *Delerium tremens* and dream deprivation. *Association for the Psychophysiological Study of Sleep*, Palo Alto, 1964.

Gresham, S. C., Webb, W. B., and Williams, R. L., Alcohol and caffeine: effects on inferred visual dreaming. *Science* 140:1226, 1963.

Gross, M. M., Goodenough, D. R., Tobin, M., Halpert, E., Dominick, L., Perlstein, A., Sirota, M., DiBianco, J., Fuller, R., and Kishner, I., Sleep disturbances and hallucinations in the acute alcoholic psychosis. *Association for the Psychophysiological Study of Sleep*, Palo Alto, 1964.

Gross, M., Goodenough, D., Baekeland, F. *et al.*, An experiment of the effects of alcohol on the sleep of alcoholics. *Association for the Psychophysiological Study of Sleep*, Palo Alto, 1966.

Halberg, F., and Howard, R. B., Twenty-four hour periodicity and experimental medicine. *Post Graduate Medicine* 24:349–358, 1958.

Hall, C. S., *The Meaning of Dreams*. New York: Dell, 1959.

Hall, C. S., and Van de Castle, R. L., A comparison of home

and monitored dreams. *Association for the Psychophysiological Study of Sleep*, Palo Alto, 1964.

Hammack, J. T., An experimental analysis of behavior during sleep. Three annual progress reports to the defense documentation center, 1962, 1963, 1964.

Hammack, J. T., Williams, J. M., Weisberg, P., Brooks, P., and Gerard, M., An experimental analysis of behavior during sleep. U.S. Army Medical Research and Development Command, 1964. Contract No. Da-49-193-MD-2180.

Hanretta, A. G., Diagnostic utilization of sleep characteristics. *Texas State Journal of Medicine* 59, September, 1963.

Harms, E. (ed.), *Problems of Sleep and Dreams in Children*, International Series of Monographs on Child Psychiatry, vol. 2, New York: Macmillan, 1964.

Hartmann, E., Pharmacological studies on man: phenobarbital (Nembutal), amitriptyline (Elavil), chlordiazepoxide (Librium) and RO 5-6901 (Dalmane). *Association for the Psychophysiological Study of Sleep*, 1967.

———, Dreaming sleep (the D-state) and the menstrual cycle. *Journal of Mental Disorders* 143:406–416, November, 1966.

———, The effect of tryptophane on the sleep-dream cycle in man. *Psychonomic Science* 8:479–480, 1967.

———, The sleep-dream cycle and brain serotonin. *Psychonomic Science* 8(7):295–296, 1967.

———, Dreaming sleep and the menstrual cycle. *Association for the Psychophysiological Study of Sleep*, Washington, D.C., 1965.

———, The D-state. *New England Journal of Medicine* 283:30, 1965.

Hauri, P., Effects of evening activity on early night sleep. *Psychophysiology* 4, 1968.

Hawkins, D. R., A review of psychoanalytic dream theory

in the light of recent psychophysiological studies of sleep and dreaming. *British Journal of Medical Psychology* 39, 1966.

Hawkins, D. R., Scott, J., and Thrasher, G., Sleep patterns in enuretic children. *Association for the Psychophysiological Study of Sleep*, Washington, D.C., 1965.

Hernandez-Peon, R., Attention, sleep, motivation and behavior. In *The Role of Pleasure in Behavior*, ed. R. Health. New York: Hoeber-Harper, 1964.

Hernandez-Peon, R., and Chavez-Ibarra, G., Sleep induced by electrical or chemical stimulation of the forebrain. *EEG Clinical Neurophysiology*, Supplement 24, 1962.

Hilgard, E. R., *Theories of Learning*. New York: Appleton-Century-Crofts, 1956.

Hobson, J. S., Sleep as a response: effects of the exercise on subsequent sleep. *Association for the Psychophysiological Study of Sleep*, 1967, 1968.

Hollander, B., *Methods and Uses of Hypnosis and Self-Hypnosis*. Hollywood, Cal.: Wilshire Book Co., 1957.

Hull, C. L., *Principles of Behavior*. New York: Appleton-Century-Crofts, 1943.

Hunter, I. M. L., *Memory, Facts and Fallacies*. Baltimore: Penguin Books, 1957.

Hyden, H., and Lange, P. W., Rhythmic enzyme changes in neurons and glia during sleep. *Science* 149:654, 1965.

Jacobson, A., Kales, A., Lehmann, D., and Hoedemaker, F. S., Muscle tonus in human subjects during sleep and dreaming. *Experimental Neurology* 10:418–424, 1964.

Jacobson, E., *Progressive Relaxation*. Chicago: Univ. of Chicago Press, 1938.

———, *You Can Sleep Well*. New York: Whittlesey House, 1938.

———, *You Must Relax*. New York: Whittlesey House, 1942.

Jeanneret, P. R., and Webb, W. B., Strength of grip on

arousal from a full night's sleep. *Perception Motor Skills* 17:759, 1963.

Johnson, L. C., Sleep and sleep loss—their effect on performance. *Naval Research*, August, 1967.

Jouvet, M., Paradoxical sleep—a study of its nature and mechanisms. In *Sleep Mechanisms*, vol. 18, eds. K. Akert, C. Bally, and J. P. Schade. Amsterdam: Elsevier Publ. Co., 1965.

Jung, C. G., "Freud and Psychoanalysis." In *The Collected Works of C. G. Jung*, vol. 4, New York: Pantheon, 1961.

Kahn, E., Dement, W. C., Fisher, C., and Barmack, J., Incidence of color in immediately recalled dreams. *Science* 137:1054, 1962.

Kales, A., and Berger, R. J., Psychopathology of sleep. In *Symptoms of Psychopathology*, ed. C. G. Costello, New York: John Wiley & Sons, 1968.

Kales, A., Jacobson, A., Marusak, C., and Hanley, J., Effects of drugs on sleep. *Association for the Psychophysiological Study of Sleep*, 1968.

Kales, A., Kales, J. D., Walter, R. D., Jacobson, A., Paulson, M. J., Recall studies in children. *Association for the Psychophysiological Study of Sleep*, 1966.

Kales, A., Wilson, T., Kales, J. D., Jacobson, A., Paulson, M. J., Kollar, E., and Walter, R. D., Measurements of all-night sleep in normal elderly persons: effects of aging. *Journal of American Geriatric Society* 15(5): 405, 1967.

Kales, A., *et al.*, Sleep and dreams. *Annals of Internal Medicine* 68(5): May, 1968.

Kamiya, J., Behavioral, subjective, and physiological aspects of drowsiness and sleep. In *Functions of Varied Experience*, eds. D. W. Fiske and S. R. Maddi, Homewood, Ill.: Dorsey, 1961.

Kaplan, J., Sleepwalking: Fact, fallacy, or fancy? *Today's Health*, September, 1960.

Karacan, I., The effect of exciting presleep events on dream reporting and penile erections during sleep. Unpublished thesis, Psychiatry Department, State University of New York, Downstate Medical Center, Brooklyn, 1965.

Karacan, I., Goodenough, D. R., Shapiro, A., and Witkin, H. A., Some psychological and physiological correlates of penile erections during sleep. *Association for the Psychophysiological Study of Sleep*, Washington, D.C., 1965.

Karacan, I., Wolff, S. M., Webb, W. B., and Williams, R. L., The effect of fever on sleep patterns. *Association for the Psychophysiological Study of Sleep*, 1968.

Kety, S. S., A biologist examines the mind and behavior. *Science* 132:1861, 1960.

Kleitman, N., *Sleep and Wakefulness* (rev. ed.). Chicago: Univ. of Chicago Press, 1963.

Koella, W. P., Trunca, C. M., and Czicman, J. S., Serotonin: effect on recruiting responses of the cat. *Life Science* 4:173–181, 1965.

Koella, W. P., and Czicman, J. S., Influence of serotonin upon optic evoked potentials, EEG, and blood pressure of cat. *American Journal of Physiology* 204:873, 1963.

Laing, A. M., *The Sleep Book*. London: Frederick Muller Ltd., 1948.

Levant, O., *Memoirs of an Amnesiac*. New York: Putnam, 1965.

Levitt, R. A., Sleep as a conditioned response. *Psychological Science* 1:273–274, 1964.

Lewin, B. D., *The Psychoanalysis of Elation*. New York: Norton, 1950.

Lewis, H. E., and Masterton, J. P., British North Greenland expedition 1952–1954. *The Lancet*, September 3 and 10, 1955.

Liberson, W. T., and Liberson, C. W., EEG, reaction time, eye movements, respiration, and mental content during drowsiness. *Association for the Psychophysiological Study of Sleep,* Washington, D.C., 1965.

Luce, G. G., and Segal, J., When children sleep. *Redbook,* January, 1967.

Marshall, S. L. A., *Night Drop.* Boston: Little, Brown, 1962.

McCann, H. W., The strange world of sleepless people. *Science Digest,* February, 1962.

Meier, G. W., and Berger, R. J., The development of sleep and wakefulness patterns in the infant Rhesus monkey. *Experimental Neurology* 12:257, 1965.

Mendels, J., and Hawkins, D. R., The psychophysiology of sleep in depression. *Mental Hygiene,* 51(4), October, 1967.

———, Sleep laboratory adaptation in normal subjects and depressed patients (first night effect). *Electroencephalography and Clinical Neurophysiology,* 22, 1967.

Metz, B., Scharf, G., and Gridel, F., Psychophysiological effects of sleep deprivation. 16th International Congress in Psychology, Bonn, Germany, 1960.

Mintz, M., *The Therapeutic Nightmare,* Boston: Houghton Mifflin, Co., 1965.

Monroe, L., Psychological and physiological differences between good and poor sleepers. *Journal of Abnormal Psychology* 72:255–264, 1967.

Moruzzi, G., The physiology of sleep. *Endeavour* 22:31–36, 1963.

———, Active processes of brain stem during sleep. *The Harvey Lecture Series,* 58, Academic Press, 1962.

Murray, E., *Sleep, Dreams and Arousal.* New York: Appleton-Century-Crofts, 1965.

Murray, E., Schein, E. H., Erickson, K. T., Hill, W. F., and Cohen, M., The effects of sleep deprivation on social behavior. *Journal of Social Psychology* 49:229, 1959.

Murray, E., Williams, H. L., and Lubin, A., Body temperature and psychological ratings during sleep deprivation. *Journal of Experimental Psychology* 56(3), September, 1958.

Newman, A. S., Sleep and the soldier. *Army*, October, 1963.

Oswald, I., *Sleeping and Waking*. New York: American Elsevier, 1962.

———, The experimental study of sleep. *British Medical Bulletin* 20:1, 1964.

———, *Sleep*. Middlesex, England: Penguin Books, 1966.

Oswald, I., and Priest, R. G., Abnormal sleep after withdrawal of hypnotics. In *Recent Advances in Biological Psychiatry*, vol. 8, ed. Wortis, New York: Plenum Press, 1966.

Parmalee, A. H., Sleep patterns in infancy. *Acta Paediatrica* 50:150–170, 1961.

Parmalee, A. H., and Wenner, W. H., Sleep states in premature and full term newborn infants. Association for the Psychophysiological Study of Sleep, Washington, D.C., 1965.

Phipps, J., and Robinson, R., The growing menace of "nice" drugs. *Good Housekeeping*, September, 1963.

Portnoff, G., Baekland, F., Goodenough, D. R., Karacan, I., and Shapiro, A., The effect of sleep on retention. Association for the Psychophysiological Study of Sleep, Washington, D.C., 1965.

Powers, M., *Hypnotism Revealed*. Hollywood, Cal.: Wilshire Book Co., 1952.

Proceedings, White House Conference on Narcotic and Drug Abuse. Gov't. Printing Office, Washington, D.C., 1962.

Rechtschaffen, A., Dream reports and dream experiences. UCLA Conf., Physiological Correlates of Dreaming, October, 1966.

Rechtschaffen, A., and Maron, L., The effect of amphetamine on the sleep cycle. *EEG Clinical Neurophysiology* 16:433–445, 1964.

Reding, G. R., Rubright, W. C., Rechtschaffen, A., and

Daniels, R. S., Sleep pattern of tooth-grinding: its relationship to dreaming. *Science* 145:725, 1964.

Reinberg, A., and Ghata, J., *Biological Rhythms*. New York: Walker & Co., 1964.

Reinhold, R., Scientists studying the sleep patterns in Antarctica, *The New York Times*, January 11, 1968.

Richter, C. P., *Biological Clocks in Medicine and Psychiatry*. Charles C. Thomas, 1965.

Roffwarg, H. P., and Fisher, C., Preliminary observations on the sleep-dream patterns of neonates, infants, children and adults. In *Problems of Sleep and Dreams in Children*, ed. E. Harms, London: Pergamon, 1963.

———, Preliminary observations on the sleep-dream patterns of neonates, infants, children and adults. In *Behavior in Infancy and Early Childhood*, eds. Y. Brackbill and C. G. Thompson, New York: The Free Press, pp. 47–60, 1967.

Rosenteur, P., *Morpheus and Me*. New York: Funk and Wagnalls, 1957.

Rossi, G. F., Sleep-inducing mechanisms in the brain stem. *EEG Clinical Neurophysiology*. Sup. 24:133–134, 1963.

———, Psychological effects of deprivation of dreaming sleep. *Journal of Nervous Mental Disorders* 143:305–317, 1966.

Schwartz, B. A., Gilbaud, G., and Fischgold, H., Sleep and insomnia. *Journal Medicale de France*, p. 127, Nancy, France, 1962.

Simon, C. W., and Emmons, W. H., Responses to material presented during various levels of sleep. *Journal of Experimental Psychology* 51:89–97, 1956.

———, Some immediate effects of drowsiness and sleep on normal human performance. *Human Factors* 3: 1961.

———, Learning during sleep. *Psychological Bulletin* 52:328–342, 1955.

———, EEG, consciousness, and sleep. *Science* 124:1066–1069, 1956.

Sleep and Altered States of Consciousness, Association for Research in Nervous and Mental Disease (45th Annual Meeting), in press.

Snyder, F., The REM state in a living fossil. *Association for the Psychophysiological Study of Sleep*, Palo Alto, 1964.

Snyder, S. H., and Axelrod, J., Circadian rhythm in pineal serotonin: effect of mono amine oxidase inhibition and reserpine. *Science* 149:542, 1965.

Svoard, D., and Novakova, V., Effect of experimentally induced insomnia in neurotic states in rats. *Fiziol. Zh. SSR, Sechenov*, 46:57–63, 1960.

Svyadoshch, A. M., Perception and memory of speech during natural sleep. *Voprosy Psikhologii* 1(1), No. 3-9-64, Trans. Unit. NIH, 1962.

Takano, R., Developmental study of nocturnal sleep. *Folia Psychiatrica Neurologica Japanes* 20(2):208–209, 1966.

Thorpe, L. P., and Schmuller, A. M., *Contemporary Theories of Learning*. New York: The Ronald Press Co., 1954.

Toxicants Occurring Naturally in Foods, Publication 1354, National Academy of Sciences, National Research Council, 1966.

Trillin, C., A third state of existence, *The New Yorker*, September 18, 1965.

Tune, G., When man doth sleep, *The New Scientist*, June 2, 1967.

Turnbow, A. W., *Sleep-Learning, Its Theory, Application and Technique*. Olympia, Wash.: Sleep-Learning Research Association, 1958.

Wagner, A. E., An experiment to determine the number of repetitions necessary to memorize and retain with maximum certainty a miscellaneous collection of facts. May, 1910.

——, Antecedents of sleep. *Journal of Experimental Psychology* 53:162, 1957.

———, The results of continued partial sleep deprivation. *Association for the Psychophysiological Study of Sleep*, Washington, D.C., 1965.

———, Sleep deprivation: age and exhaustion time in the rat. *Science* 136:1122, 1962.

Weiss, T., and Roldan, E., Comparative study of sleep cycles in rodents. *Experientia* 20:280–281, 1964.

Weitzman, E. D., and Kremen, H., Auditory evoked responses during different stages of sleep in man. *EEG Clinical Neurophysiology* 18:65–70, 1965.

West, L. J., United States Air Force prisoners of Chinese communists. In Methods of Forceful Indoctrination: Observations and Interviews, *Group for the Advancement of Psychiatry Symposium* 4:270–284, 1957.

Whitman, R. M., Pierce, C., Maas, J., and Baldridge, B., The dreams of the experimental subject. *Journal of Nervous Mental Disorders* 134:431–439, 1962.

Wilkinson, R. T., Effects of up to 60 hours of sleep deprivation on different types of work. *Ergonontics* 7:175–186, 1964.

———, After-effect of sleep deprivation. *Journal of Experimental Psychology* 66:439–444, 1963.

———, Interaction of noise with knowledge of results and sleep deprivation. *Journal of Experimental Psychology* 66:332–337, 1963.

———, Sleep deprivation. In *Physiology of Survival*. New York: Academic Press, 1966.

Williams, H. L., Sleep starvation and you. *Army Information Digest*, June, 1964.

Williams, H. L., Lester, B. K., and Coulte, J. D., Monoamines and the EEG stages of sleep. *Association for the Psychophysiological Study of Sleep*, Palo Alto, 1968.

Williams, H. L., Lubin, A., and Goodnow, J. J., Impaired performance with acute sleep loss. *Psychological Monograph* No. 484, 73(14), 1959, Am. Psychol. Assn., Washington, D.C.

Williams, H. L., *et al.*, Sleep patterns in young adults: an EEG study. *EEG Clinical Neurophysiology* 17:376–381, 1964.

Wilson, W. P., and Zung, W. K., Arousal threshold of males and females during sleep. 10th Ann. Conf. V.A. Cooperative Studies in Psychiatry, New Orleans, La., March, 1965.

Witkin, H. A., and Lewis, H. B., The relation of experimentally induced pre-sleep experiences to dreams: a report of methods and preliminary findings. *Journal of American Psychoanalytic Association*, October, 1965.

Wolf, W. (ed.), Rhythmic functions in the living system. *Annals of the New York Academy of Sciences* 98(4), October, 1962.

Wolstenholme, G. E. W., and O'Connor, M. (eds.), *The Nature of Sleep*. Boston: Little, Brown, 1960.

Wood, P. B., Dreaming and social isolation. Unpublished Ph.D. dissertation, Univ. of North Carolina, 1962.

Woods, R. L., *The World of Dreams*. New York: Random House, 1947.

Yogananda, P., *Autobiography of a Yogi*. Self-Realization Fellowship, Los Angeles, 1959.

Zimmerman, W. B., Psychological and physiological differences between "light" and "deep" sleepers. Ph.D. dissertation, University of Chicago, September, 1967.

Zung, W. G., and Wilson, W. P., Sleep and dream patterns in twins: Markov chain analysis of a genetic trait. In *Recent Advances in Biological Psychiatry* 9:119–30, Plenum Press, 1967.

OTHER SELECTIONS FROM PLAYBOY PRESS

MARRIAGE CONFIDENTIAL $1.75
JEFFREY FEINMAN
An inside look at unusual and shocking weddings and marriages the world over.

HOW TO GET THE MOST FOR
YOUR MEDICAL DOLLAR $1.95
JORDAN C. LEWIS
The complete insider's guide to saving money on your health, medical and dental bills.

HOW TO WIN! SWEEPSTAKES, CONTESTS,
LOTTERIES AND BINGO $1.50
JEFFREY FEINMAN
An expert shows you how to improve the odds and be a winner.

WHAT UNCLE SAM OWES YOU $1.95
JEFFREY FEINMAN
A guide to cashing in on government giveaways, benefits and services.

est: THE MOVEMENT AND THE MAN $1.95
PAT R. MARKS
All about Erhard Seminars Training—the four-day mind game that has 60,000 graduates—and the man, Werner Erhard, who created, organized and runs it.

Order directly from:

Playboy Press
The Playboy Building
919 North Michigan Avenue
Chicago, Illinois 60611

No. of copies		Title	Pri
_____	K16337	Marriage Confidential	$1.
_____	E16324	How to Get the Most for Your Medical Dollar	$1.
_____	C16319	How to Win! Sweepstakes, Contests, Lotteries and Bingo	$1.
_____	E16304	What Uncle Sam Owes You	$1.
_____	E16317	est: The Movement and the Man	$1.

Please enclose 50¢ for postage and handling.

Total amount enclosed: $_____

Name _____

Address _____

City _____ State _____ Zip _____